First Aid
or Babies
nd Children *fast*

In association with **BritishRedCross**

First Aid
for Babies
and Children *fast*

Chief Medical Adviser: British Red Cross
Dr Vivien J Armstrong

LONDON, NEW YORK, MUNICH, MELBOURNE, DELHI

COOLING BROWN
Art Director Arthur Brown
Editor Jemima Dunne
Design Peter Cooling, Tish Jones

DORLING KINDERSLEY LIMITED
Managing Editor Penny Warren
Managing Art Editor Marianne Markham
Senior Art Editor Glenda Fisher
Jacket Designer Neal Cobourne
DTP Designer Sonia Charbonnier
Production Maria Elia
Additional photography Gary Ombler, Dave King

First published in Great Britain as First Aid for Children Fast in 1994; revised in 1999 and 2002
This fourth revision published 2006 by Dorling Kindersley Limited,
80 Strand, London WC2R 0RL

A Penguin Company
2 4 6 8 10 9 7 5 3 1

A CIP catalogue record for this book is available from the British Library

ISBN 13: 978-1-4053-1144-1
ISBN 10: 1-4053-1144-4

Reproduced in Italy by GRB
Printed and bound in Singapore by Tien Wah Press

Discover more at
www.dk.com

Foreword

Children are naturally adventurous and everyone recognises that accidents and injuries are all part of growing up. Fortunately most injuries are minor and children recover quickly but sometimes help is needed and in serious incidents it is important that a child receives the best possible initial care. In recent times there has been an increasing awareness of the importance of immediate care or first aid. There is no doubt that the right care can preserve life and speed up a child's recovery.

This revised edition of *First Aid for Babies and Children Fast* has been produced to include the latest guidelines for life-saving procedures and will bring you up to date with changes in first aid in response to new clinical evidence and modern technology. This book includes the most up-to-date rescuscitation guidelines for children and new information on protocols for the use of a defibrillator, a machine that can, in some circumstances, restart a child's heart. There are also expanded sections on important childhood conditions such as asthma, meningitis, and severe allergic reaction, or anaphylactic shock.

I hope that this book will add to and update your first aid skills and contribute to your ability to care for your injured or ill child.

Dr Vivien J Armstrong MBBS FRCA DRCOG PGCE (FE)
Chief Medical Adviser to the British Red Cross

Contents

Introduction

This book has been compiled primarily for parents but also for others – grandparents, teachers, childminders, playgroup leaders, and babysitters – who may regularly, or even occasionally, find themselves in charge of infants and children. The content has been set out in a clear and logical way and the information presented largely in pictorial form using simple words and captions to make it very easy to follow and to understand. The first aid techniques described reflect the relevant guidance set out by the Paediatric Life Support Group of the European Resuscitation Council and are current at the time of publication. They can be used to treat any age child up to puberty.

Emergencies are, by their very nature, unexpected events and require a prompt and proper response. If you follow the advice and guidance given in this book you will undoubtedly be able to give early and effective help whenever it is needed. You should be aware, however, that first aid is essentially a practical skill and your confidence and effectiveness will be greatly enhanced by expert training in a practical setting. The British Red Cross regularly runs a wide variety of first aid learning programmes, some exclusively concerned with first aid for young children. You can find out more about these by ringing your local British Red Cross office, the number is in your phone book, call 0870 170 7000, or visit www.redcross.org.uk.

Giving first aid – coping with the emergency and doing the right thing early and effectively – can be straightforward, but it can also be stressful, sometimes distasteful (especially if the child is not your own), and even dangerous. It is important that you remain in control of your feelings and avoid any tendency to rash action that could result in additional harm to an injured child or to yourself. You cannot give effective help if you yourself become a casualty so you must always take a little time to think before you act. This book is intended to help you to do the right thing at the right time – safely and effectively.

How to use this book

This book covers first aid treatment for everything from minor cuts and grazes to treating an unconscious child. For every condition a series of photographs shows you exactly what to do in an emergency. Key pieces of information are indicated on the photographs and supplementary advice can be found alongside in the step-by-step text.

The injuries are organised by type, in coloured sections such as Wounds and Bleeding and Bites and Stings. However, in an emergency, the thumbnail index on the back cover will direct you straight to the relevant page. There are also sections, such as Action in an Emergency, Bandages and Dressings, and Home Safety, that contain information for general reference.

Key signs and symptoms help you to recognise the conditions

Annotations highlight essential action

Clear photographs illustrate every step of treatment

Important boxes draw attention to areas of concern

Symbols highlight the action necessary for medical help

Cross-references direct you to pages with information about associated injuries

GUIDE TO THE SYMBOLS

The following symbols and instructions appear if your child needs further medical attention:

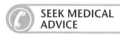

SEEK MEDICAL ADVICE

Depending on your area, call your doctor's surgery, nurse practitioner, duty paramedic, NHS direct, or the local NHS walk-in centre for advice.

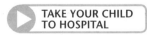

TAKE YOUR CHILD TO HOSPITAL

Take your child to the nearest accident and emergency department if you have help and transport.

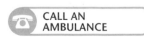

CALL AN AMBULANCE

Your child needs urgent medical attention and is best transported by ambulance to hospital.

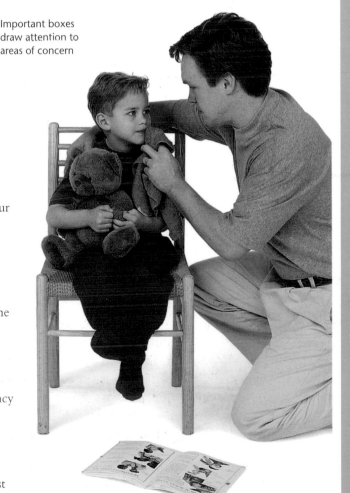

Action in an emergency

In any emergency, particularly one involving children, it is important to keep calm and act logically. Remember four steps:

1 Assess the situation

- What happened?
- How did it happen?
- Is there more than one injured child?
- Is there any continuing danger?
- Is there anyone who can help?
- Do I need an ambulance?

2 Think of safety

- Do not risk injuring yourself – you cannot help if you become a casualty.
- Remove any source of danger from your child.
- Move your child only if you must for her safety and do so very carefully.

3 Treat serious injuries first

In children, there are two conditions that immediately threaten life:
- Inability to breathe (see UNCONSCIOUSNESS p. 14).
- Serious bleeding – this is usually obvious and can be brought under control (see p. 44).

> **! IMPORTANT**
> - If more than one child is injured go quickly to the quiet one – she may be unconscious.

4 Get help

Shout for help early and ask others to:
- Make the area safe.
- Seek medical advice or call an ambulance.
- Help with first aid.
- Move a child to safety, if necessary.

Telephoning for help

When you call the emergency services, ask for an ambulance and give the following information:
- Your telephone number.
- The location of the incident.
- The type of incident.
- The number, sex, and ages of the casualties.
- Details of injuries.
- Information about hazards such as gas, power lines, or fog.

Fire

Write down an escape plan for your home and make sure everyone knows what to do.
- How would you get out of each room?
- How do you help babies and young children?
- Where will you meet when you've escaped?

Action for a chip pan fire

- Turn off stove or hob, then cover pan with lid, wet tea towel, or fire blanket – leave this on for half an hour – NEVER throw water over the flames.
- If fire is not under control, get out of the house, closing doors behind you, and call the fire brigade.

Escaping from a fire

1 Feel the door. If the door is cool, leave the room.

OR

2 If the door is hot, don't open it. Go to the window.

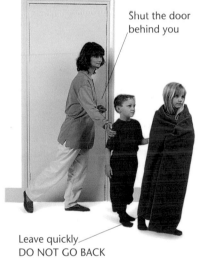

Shut the door behind you

Leave quickly
DO NOT GO BACK

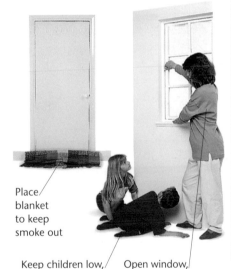

Place blanket to keep smoke out

Keep children low, where air is clearest

Open window, call for help

! IMPORTANT

- **Carry** babies and toddlers.
- **Don't** ask children to do anything other than look after themselves.
- **Close** all doors behind you.
- **Meet** outside your house.
- **Never** go back inside.
- **Phone** for help from elsewhere.

If you have to escape through a window

- **Slide** your child out, hang onto him, then ask him to drop down.
- **Slide** out yourself, hang from the ledge, then drop.
- **If** you have to break the glass first, put a blanket over the frame before you escape.

Clothing on fire

If clothing is on fire:
Stop your child moving as movement will fan the flames.
Drop him to the floor to stop him burning his face and airway.
Wrap him in a coat or blanket to help smother the flames.
Roll him on the ground.

! IMPORTANT

- **Do not** let your child run about in a panic; rapid movement will fan the flames.
- **If** water is available, lay him down, burning side uppermost, and douse him with water or a non-flammable liquid.

! IMPORTANT

● **Never** touch your child's skin. Pull at his clothes as a last resort.

● **If your child is unconscious**, open his airway and check breathing. If breathing, place in the recovery position; if not breathing, begin rescue breaths and chest compressions.

High-voltage current

Contact with electricity from power lines and overhead cables is usually fatal. Severe burns result and the child may be thrown some distance from the point of contact. NEVER approach the child unless you know for sure that the power has been cut off.

» *see also*

● Electrical burns, *p.60*

● Unconscious baby, *pp.17–21*

● Unconscious child, *pp.22–29*

Electrical injury

Children are at risk of electric shock if they play with electrical sockets or flexes. Electrical current causes muscle spasms that prevent a child letting go of an electric cable and may cause burns both where it enters and leaves the child's body. If an electrical current passes through a child's body, it may also cause breathing and heart to stop.

Stand on insulating material

Push the source away

Wrap a dry towel around his feet

☎ CALL AN AMBULANCE

1 Break the contact with electricity by switching the current off at the mains.

2 If you cannot switch off the current, stand on dry insulating material such as telephone books or a wooden box. Use a wooden broom handle or chair to separate your child's limbs from the source.

3 If you still cannot break the contact without touching your child, wrap a dry towel around his feet and pull him away from the source.

4 When the contact is broken, treat any injuries. If the child seems unharmed, make him rest and observe his condition.

Drowning

Babies and young children can drown quickly if they slip into a pool or pond or are left unattended in a bath. Even 2.5cm (1in) of water is enough to cover a baby's nose and mouth if she falls forwards.

Keep her head lower than her chest

1 Lift your child out of the water. Carry her with her head lower than her chest to reduce the risk of inhaling water.

2 Remove any wet clothing and cover her with a dry towel or blanket.

3 If your child is unconscious, open the airway and check breathing. If breathing, place her in the recovery position; if she is not breathing, begin rescue breaths and chest compressions.

☎ **CALL AN AMBULANCE**

! IMPORTANT

● **If** you need to give rescue breaths you may need to blow into the child's mouth more firmly and more slowly than usual to get the chest to rise. Water and the effects of cold can increase resistance to rescue breathing.

● **Always** seek medical advice even if she appears to have recovered. She may have inhaled some water, which can cause lung damage.

Rescue in open water

A child may get into difficulty in open water especially if it is turbulent or very cold. Rescue her quickly. Try to reach her from the shore or bank with your hand, or with a stick. Get her dry and warm as quickly as possible.

» *see also*
● Hypothermia, *p.90*
● Unconscious baby, *pp.17–21*
● Unconscious child, *pp.22–29*

Unconsciousness

A baby or child needs to inhale oxygen into their lungs. This oxygen passes into the bloodstream and is pumped around the body by the heart. If a baby or child is unconscious, the airway to the lungs may be blocked so oxygen can't enter the body. Lack of oxygen slows down the heartbeat until it stops (cardiac arrest) and no oxygen will reach the brain.

What you can do

If a child is unconscious, you must open the airway. Then, if necessary, breathe into the lungs (rescue breathing). If circulation stops, oxygenated blood cannot travel to the brain so you need to drive the blood to the brain with chest compressions. This is known as cardiopulmonary resuscitation (CPR). A machine called a defibrillator can be used to restore a normal heartbeat in a child over the age of one (*see p.23*).

Always make sure it is safe to approach the baby or child; you can't help if you become a casualty too. When you are certain you are safe, assess whether he or she is conscious, then follow the ABC of resuscitation: A for airway, B for Breathing and C for Compressions.

Chain of survival

An unconscious baby or child's chances of survival are greater if:

- You call for expert help;
- CPR is given as soon as possible;
- A defibrillator is used early;
- Advanced care by paramedics and hospital is received as soon as possible.

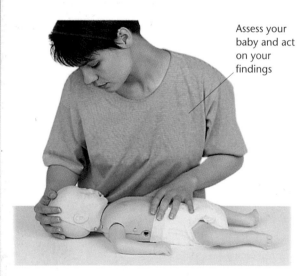

Assess your baby and act on your findings

Assess your child and act on your findings

Tap his shoulder

A is for airway

You need to open the air passage, or airway. Place one hand on the forehead and gently tilt the head back to bring the tongue away from the back of the throat. If you suspect a neck injury, use the jaw thrust method to open the airway (*see p. 70*).

Airway

If child is on his back the tongue falls back and blocks the airway.

Tongue fallen back

Blocked airway – head not tilted

Tongue forward

Unblocked airway – head tilted

For a baby

Tilt the head back to clear the airway

For a child

Tilt the head back to clear the airway

B is for breathing

If your child is not breathing after the airway has been opened, take a breath and blow steadily into the lungs to get oxygen into the child's blood.

For a baby

Blow into the mouth and nose until the chest rises

For a child

Hold the nose and blow into the mouth

C is for compressions

If your child's heart has stopped giving chest compressions will drive blood containing oxygen around the body. This is always combined with rescue breathing. The combination of techniques is known as cardiopulmonary resuscitation (CPR).

For a baby

For a child

Press on centre of the chest with two fingers

Press on centre of the chest with one hand

When to call an ambulance

If there is somebody else present to help, always ask him or her to call an ambulance as soon as you realise that your child is not breathing. If you are on your own, give rescue breaths (*see* rescue breathing: baby *p.18*; child *p.24*) and chest compressions (*see* CPR: baby *p.20*; child *p.26*), for 1 minute before pausing to CALL AN AMBULANCE.

Unconscious baby

Assess your baby before calling for help. If you are alone and the baby is not breathing, begin rescue breaths and chest compressions.

1 Check for response

- Call her name, or tap her foot gently. Never shake a baby.
- If there is no response, continue to step 2.
- If there is a reponse,

SEEK MEDICAL ADVICE

Call her name

2 Open baby's airway

- Put one hand on the baby's forehead and gently tilt her head.
- Place one finger of your other hand on the tip of her chin and lift it.

! IMPORTANT
- **Do not** press on the soft part of the neck as it can block the airway.

Tilt head back
Lift chin with one finger

3 Check breathing for up to 10 seconds

- Look, listen, and feel for breathing. Look along her chest for movement, listen for sounds of normal breathing, and feel for breaths against your cheek. Send helper to:

CALL AN AMBULANCE

- If she is breathing, hold her with head down and wait for help.
- If she not breathing give five initial rescue breaths – GO TO PAGE 18.

Listen for breaths
Look for chest movements
Feel for breath on your cheek

Resuscitation summary

Unconscious baby

Airway open

No breathing

Send helper to

CALL AN AMBULANCE

Give five initial rescue breaths

Begin chest compressions with rescue breaths (CPR)

Repeat for 1 minute

If not already done,

CALL AN AMBULANCE

Continue CPR until help arrives

Resuscitation summary

Unconscious baby

Airway open

No breathing

Send helper to

 CALL AN AMBULANCE

Give five initial rescue breaths

Begin chest compressions with rescue breaths (CPR)

Repeat for 1 minute

If not already done,

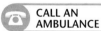 **CALL AN AMBULANCE**

Continue CPR until help arrives

Rescue breathing: baby

This is to be used for an unconscious baby who is not breathing. Always give five initial rescue breaths before beginning chest compressions.

Tilt head back

Lift point of chin with one finger

1 · Make sure your baby is on her back on a firm surface. Check that her airway is open. Place your fingers on the point of the chin. Don't press on the soft tissues under the chin as you could block the airway. Lift her chin.

Pick out visible obstructions

2 Pick out any visible obstruction from the mouth and nose with your fingertips, but do not do a finger sweep.

Breathe into the baby's mouth and nose

3 Take a breath, then seal your lips tightly around your baby's mouth and nose. Blow gently into the lungs until the chest rises.

Watch chest fall after a breath

4 Remove your mouth and watch the chest fall back.

Repeat to give five rescue breaths

5 Repeat to give five rescue breaths. If you can't achieve a rescue breath, recheck the airway, recheck the mouth and nose (remove any visible obstruction), and make sure you have a tight seal around the mouth and nose. Don't try more than five times.

Press down by one-third of the depth of the chest

6 Begin chest compressions. GO TO PAGE 20.

Resuscitation summary

Unconscious baby

Airway open

No breathing

Send helper to

☎ CALL AN AMBULANCE

Give 5 initial rescue breaths

Begin chest compressions with rescue breaths (CPR)

Repeat for 1 minute

If not already done,

☎ CALL AN AMBULANCE

Continue CPR until help arrives

CPR: baby

This is a combination of chest compressions and rescue breaths used to treat an unconscious baby who is not breathing. If you are on your own give CPR for a full minute before you call an ambulance.

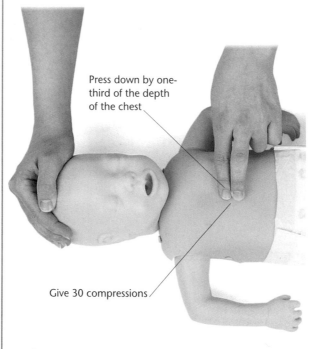

Press down by one-third of the depth of the chest

Give 30 compressions

1 Place your baby on a firm surface. Place the tips of two fingers on the centre of the baby's chest.

2 Press down sharply by one-third of the depth of the chest. Release the pressure but don't remove your fingers. Allow chest to come back up fully. Repeat to give 30 compressions at a rate of 100 per minute.

Give two rescue breaths

3 Give your baby two rescue breaths into her mouth and nose.

Repeat 30 chest compressions

Follow with two rescue breaths

Repeat 30 chest compressions

Follow with two rescue breaths

4 Continue the cycle of 30 chest compressions to two rescue breaths for 1 minute.

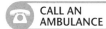 **CALL AN AMBULANCE**

5 Continue giving CPR – 30 chest compressions followed by two rescue breaths – until emergency help arrives, the baby starts breathing, or you are too exhausted to continue.

 IMPORTANT

● **If** breathing returns, cradle your baby in your arms with her head tilted down and CALL AN AMBULANCE if not already done. Monitor your baby carefully until the ambulance arrives.

● **Take** your baby with you when you go to call the ambulance.

» *see also*
● Rescue breathing: baby, *p.18*

Resuscitation summary

Unconscious child

Airway open

No breathing

Send helper to

CALL AN AMBULANCE

Give five initial rescue breaths

Begin chest compressions with rescue breaths (CPR)

Repeat for 1 minute

If not already done,

CALL AN AMBULANCE

Continue CPR until help arrives

Unconscious child

Assess your child before calling for help. If you are on your own and the child is not breathing, begin rescue breaths and chest compressions.

1 Check for response

- Call his name, or tap his shoulder gently. Never shake a child.
- If there is no response, go to step 2.
- If there is a response,

 SEEK MEDICAL ADVICE

Tap his shoulder gently

2 Open child's airway

- Put one hand on the child's forehead and gently tilt his head back.
- Place two fingers of your other hand on the tip of his chin and lift it.

! IMPORTANT
- **Do not** press on the soft part of the neck as it can block the airway.

Lift chin with two fingers

Tilt head back

3 Check breathing for up to 10 seconds

- Look, listen, and feel for breathing. Look along his chest for movement, listen for sounds of normal breathing, and feel for breaths against your cheek. Send a helper to:

 CALL AN AMBULANCE

Feel for breath on your cheek

Look for chest movements

- If he is breathing place him in the recovery position. GO TO PAGE 28.
- If he not breathing, begin rescue breaths. GO TO PAGE 24.

Using a paediatric defibrillator

Machines called automated external defibrillators (AEDs), or defibrillators, can be used to restart a child's heart. Ideally, use a special paediatric or children's defibrillator for a child between the ages of one to eight, or an adult machine with paediatric pads. An adult defibrillator can be used on a child over the age of eight (do not use defibrillators on babies under the age of one year). Always begin rescue breaths and chest compressions (*see pp. 24–27*) and follow the instructions given by the defibrillator. If the child starts breathing, leave the pads attached and place her in the recovery position (*see p. 28*).

1 Put the defibrillator beside the child, switch it on, and take out the electrode pads. Make sure they are attached to the machine.

2 Place the pads on the child's chest. Follow the instructions: peel off the backing paper and put one on the upper right side of the child's chest and the other on lower left hand side of the chest.

3 Once the pads are attached, move away from the child and make sure no-one is touching her. The defibrillator will analyse the heart and may recommend delivering a shock. Listen to the prompts given by the machine.

Place one pad on left side of chest so that long axis is vertical

Ask any helper to stay clear of the child during analysis and shock

Defibrillator

Place one pad on upper right side of chest

IF SHOCK IS ADVISED
- The defibrillator will start to charge up – make sure everyone is well clear of the child.
- Push the shock button when the defibrillator gives the instruction.
- Continue chest compressions and rescue breaths until the machine asks you to stop.
- Machine will re-analyse the child's heart rhythm.

IF SHOCK IS NOT ADVISED
- Continue chest compressions and rescue breaths until the defibrillator asks you to stop.
- Machine will re-analyse the child's heart rhythm.

Resuscitation summary

Unconscious child

Airway open

No breathing

Send helper to

 CALL AN AMBULANCE

Give five initial rescue breaths

Begin chest compressions with rescue breaths (CPR)

Repeat for 1 minute

If not already done,

 CALL AN AMBULANCE

Continue CPR until help arrives

Rescue breathing: child

This is to be used for an unconscious child who is not breathing. Always give five initial rescue breaths before beginning chest compressions.

Tilt head back to open the airway

1 Make sure that his airway is open. Place your fingers on the point of the chin. Don't press on the soft tissues under the chin, as you could block the airway. Lift the child's chin.

Remove visible obstructions from mouth

2 Pick out visible obstructions from the child's mouth with your fingertips, but do not do a finger sweep.

Take a breath and blow into the child's mouth

3 Pinch his nostrils closed. Take a breath then seal your lips round his mouth. Blow into his mouth for one second until you see the chest rise.

Watch the chest
fall after the
breath

4 Remove your
mouth and watch
the chest fall. Keep the
nostrils pinched. If your
child's chest does not
rise, check his mouth
again and adjust the
position of his head.

> **! IMPORTANT**
>
> ● **If** breathing returns,
> place your child in the
> recovery position (*see
> p.28*) and CALL AN
> AMBULANCE if not
> already done. Monitor
> him carefully until the
> ambulance arrives.

Give five rescue
breaths

5 Give five rescue
breaths. If you can't
achieve breaths after five
attempts, stop.

Begin chest
compressions

6 After five attempts
at rescue breaths,
begin chest compressions.
GO TO PAGE 26.

Resuscitation summary

Unconscious child

Airway open

No breathing

Send helper to

 CALL AN AMBULANCE

Give five initial rescue breaths

Begin chest compressions with rescue breaths (CPR)

Repeat for 1 minute

If not already done,

 CALL AN AMBULANCE

Continue CPR until help arrives

CPR: child

This is a combination of chest compressions and rescue breaths used to treat an unconscious child who is not breathing. If you are alone, give CPR for a full minute before you call an ambulance.

Place hand on centre of chest

1 Place your child on his back on a firm surface. Place the heel of your hand on the centre of the child's chest. Lean forwards over the child so your shoulder is above your hand.

Lean directly over the child and press down on the chest

2 Press down sharply by one-third of the depth of the chest. Release the pressure but don't move your hand. Let the chest come back up fully. Do this 30 times at a rate of 100 compressions per minute.

Give two
rescue breaths

3 Tilt the child's head back, lift the chin, and give TWO rescue breaths (*see p.24*).

4 Continue the CPR cycle of 30 chest compressions to two rescue breaths for 1 minute. Then if not already done,

CALL AN AMBULANCE

Repeat 30 chest compressions

5 Continue giving CPR – 30 chest compressions followed by two rescue breaths – until emergency help arrives, the child starts breathing, or you are too exhausted to continue.

! **IMPORTANT**

● **If** breathing returns, place your child in the recovery position (*see p.28*) and monitor him carefully until the ambulance arrives.

For a larger child or small rescuer

If the child is large, or you are small, you can deliver chest compressions with two hands. Place one hand on the centre of the child's chest, then place your other hand on top and interlock your fingers. Then press down with the heel of both hands.

Interlock your fingers

Keep your fingers off the child's chest

Recovery position

Put your child in this position if she is unconscious but is breathing to prevent her choking on her tongue or vomit.

Bend arm nearest to you at a right angle

1 Kneel beside your child. Remove spectacles and any bulky objects from her pockets. If necessary, straighten her legs. Bend the arm nearest to you so that it makes a right angle and lay it on the ground, with the palm of the hand upwards.

Move furthest arm across her chest and bend it

Place back of her hand against her cheek

2 Bring her other arm across her chest. Hold the back of her hand against her opposite cheek.

Clasp under thigh of outside leg and bend at knee

Place her foot flat on ground

Keep this leg straight

Support her hand against her cheek

3 Use your free hand to clasp gently under the thigh that is furthest from you. Carefully pull the knee up to bend the leg, leaving the foot flat on the ground.

4 Keep your child's hand against her cheek to support her head. At the same time, pull on the thigh of the bent leg to roll your child towards you and onto her side.

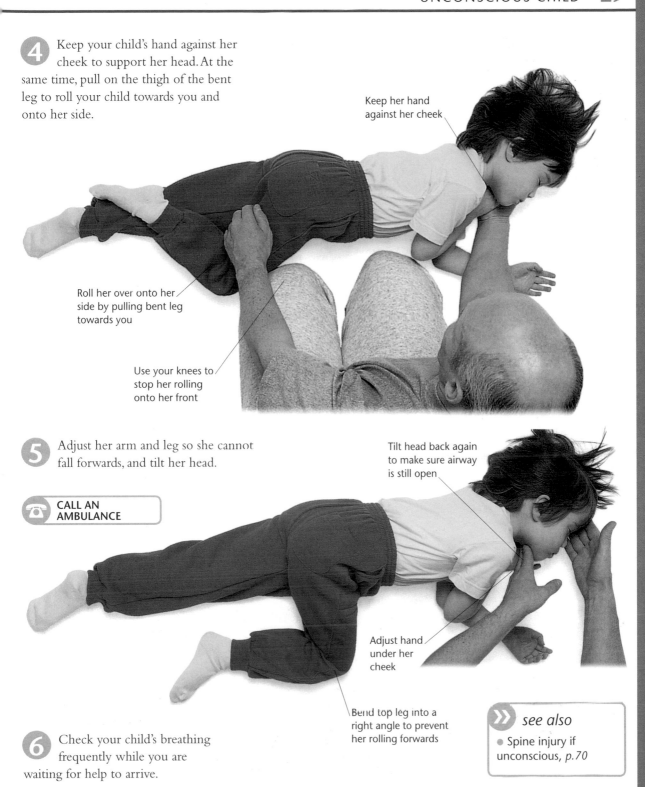

Keep her hand against her cheek

Roll her over onto her side by pulling bent leg towards you

Use your knees to stop her rolling onto her front

5 Adjust her arm and leg so she cannot fall forwards, and tilt her head.

☎ CALL AN AMBULANCE

Tilt head back again to make sure airway is still open

Adjust hand under her cheek

Bend top leg into a right angle to prevent her rolling forwards

6 Check your child's breathing frequently while you are waiting for help to arrive.

>> *see also*
• Spine injury if unconscious, *p.70*

Shock

The most likely cause of shock is serious bleeding or a severe burn or scald. These injuries must be treated without delay. There could be internal bleeding if there are signs of shock and no visible injury. Early signs are: pale, cold, and sweaty skin, tinged with grey; rapid pulse becoming weaker; shallow, fast breathing. As it develops you will notice: restlessness; yawning and sighing; severe thirst; then unconsciousness.

Help your child to lie down

Reassure him

Move child as little as possible

1 Help your child to lie down flat, on a blanket or rug if possible to protect him from the cold. Stay calm and reassure him. Treat any injury found.

☎ **CALL AN AMBULANCE**

2 Keep your child's head lower than his chest. Carefully raise your child's legs to help blood flow to the heart; support them on pillows, a chair, or a pile of books padded with a cushion.

Head must be lower than his chest

Raise his legs high above level of his heart

3 To make breathing easier, loosen any fastenings or tight clothing at his neck, chest, and waist.

4 Put a blanket or coat over your child to keep him warm. DO NOT give him a hot-water bottle or apply any other source of direct heat; it can draw blood away from the heart.

Loosen any tight clothing

Reassure your child

Cover him with a blanket

Observe and monitor his pulse, breathing rate, and level of consciousness

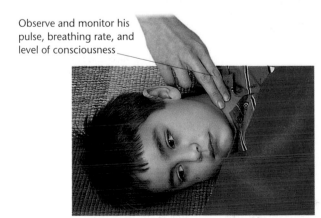

5 Monitor his pulse, breathing rate, and level of consciousness while you wait for the ambulance. Encourage him to talk or answer questions. This will help you assess any change in his condition. Note any changes and tell the ambulance personnel.

》 *see also*

● Bleeding, *p.44*

● Burns and scalds, *p.58*

● Unconscious baby, *pp.17–21*

● Unconscious child, *pp.22–29*

Febrile seizures

Young children may develop these seizures when they have a high temperature. Suspect a possible febrile seizure if: your child is flushed and sweating with a very hot forehead; her eyes are rolled upwards, and possibly fixed or squinting; she is holding her breath and her face looks blue; she stiffens, arches her back and clenches her fists.

Protect her with padding

1 Place soft padding, such as towels or pillows, around your child so that even violent movement will not lead to injury.

Cool her by removing clothing

2 Undress your child to help cool her down. Make sure there is a good supply of cool fresh air, but be careful not to overcool her.

After seizure stops, cover her with a sheet

Place her in recovery position

3 Seizures will stop when your child is cooled. Place her in the recovery position. Cover her with a light blanket or sheet and reassure her. If her temperature rises again, repeat steps 1 and 2.

SEEK MEDICAL ADVICE

» *see also*
- Fever, *p.96*
- Unconscious baby, *pp.17–21*
- Unconscious child, *pp.22–29*

Epileptic seizures

These are caused by a disturbance in the electrical activity of the brain and can be minor or major. A major seizure may progress through stages: sudden unconsciousness, sometimes with a cry; rigidity and arching of back; breathing may cease; jerking movements begin; froth or bubbles appear at the mouth, possibly blood stained; loss of bladder or bowel control. The child regains consciousness within a few minutes and appears dazed. Afterwards she may fall into a deep sleep.

Clear away nearby objects, such as chairs

Protect her head with soft padding

Place her in the recovery position if breathing

1 If your child starts to fall, help her to the floor. Prevent injury by clearing away objects that she may knock against.

2 Place padding under or around her head to prevent injury.

3 When her seizure is over, your child may be unconscious. Remove any padding and open her airway and check breathing.

4 If she is breathing, place her in the recovery position. Stay with her until she is recovered. She may feel dazed and behave oddly, or sleep deeply.

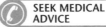 SEEK MEDICAL ADVICE

! IMPORTANT

● **Look** for a card or bracelet alerting you to the fact that a child has a history of epilepsy.

● **Do not** hold her down or try to move her during the seizure.

● **Do not** put anything in her mouth or give her anything to eat or drink.

● **If** your child has never had a seizure before, if she has repeated seizures, or if she is unconscious for more than 10 minutes CALL AN AMBULANCE.

Minor seizures

A child may have a minor seizure before a major one. This can be recognised by a momentary "switching off", some facial twitching, or distracted movements such as lip-smacking. If this happens, reassure the child and SEEK MEDICAL ADVICE.

›› *see also*

● Unconscious baby, *pp.17–21*

● Unconscious child, *pp.22–29*

Diabetic emergency

If a child with diabetes has low blood sugar levels he will be: weak or hungry; confused or behave aggressively; sweating; very pale. He may also have a strong, bounding pulse and breathing may be shallow.

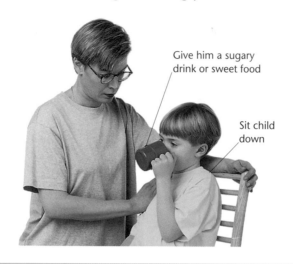

Give him a sugary drink or sweet food

Sit child down

1 Help your child to sit down and give him a sweet drink or food to raise blood sugar levels.

2 If he improves rapidly after a sweet drink or food, give him some more and let him rest.

SEEK MEDICAL ADVICE

If the child is unconscious

If a child with diabetes is unconscious, don't give her anything to eat or drink.

CALL AN AMBULANCE

1 Open the airway and check breathing.

2 If she is breathing, place her in the recovery position.

3 If she is not breathing, begin rescue breaths and chest compressions.

Open airway

Check for breathing

Place breathing child in the recovery position

Faint

Your child may be about to faint if she complains of feeling weak, giddy and sick, and is very pale. Loss of consciousness is brief and accompanied by a very slow pulse; recovery is rapid and complete.

Raise her legs above the level of her heart

Loosen any tight clothing

1 Help your child to lie down and raise her legs above the level of her heart; this improves the blood flow to her brain. Support her legs on a pile of cushions or folded blankets. Loosen any tight clothing around her neck, chest, or waist.

2 Give her plenty of fresh air. If you are inside open a window. It can help to fan her face to circulate the air. Reassure your child and help her to sit her up gradually.

SEEK MEDICAL ADVICE

Cool her by fanning her face

! IMPORTANT

● **If** child is unconscious, open her airway and check breathing. If breathing, place in the recovery position; if not breathing, begin rescue breaths and chest compressions. CALL AN AMBULANCE.

Slow recovery

Place her in the recovery position if she is slow to regain consciousness. SEEK MEDICAL ADVICE.

» see also

● Unconscious child, pp.22–29

Choking baby

If the choking is mild, your baby will still be able to cough, and cry. If the blockage is severe, however, he will be unable to cry, cough, or breathe. Give back blows then chest thrusts to relieve the blockage.

Lay him along your forearm

Give five sharp blows on his back with heel of hand

Keep his head low

Turn him onto his back

Look in mouth and remove visible object

Give five sharp downwards chest thrusts

Place two fingers on breastbone, just the below the line between the nipples

1 If your baby is unable to cough or breathe, lay him face down, head low, along your forearm. Support his head and shoulders with your hand. Give five sharp blows to the upper part of his back with the heel of your hand.

2 Turn him face up along your other arm. Look inside his mouth and pick out any visible obstruction from the mouth or nose with your forefinger and thumb.

3 If back blows fail, give chest thrusts. Place two fingers on the lower half of the baby's breastbone and give five sharp downwards thrusts at a rate of one every three seconds. Then check the baby's mouth.

4 If the blockage hasn't cleared, repeat steps 1–3 three times.

☎ **CALL AN AMBULANCE**

5 Continue cycles of back blows and chest thrusts until help arrives, the obstruction clears, or the baby loses consciousness.

If your baby becomes unconscious

If your baby loses consciousness treat as here. If he starts breathing at any stage, cradle him in your arms with his head tilted down and SEEK MEDICAL ADVICE.

Check breathing

Clear visible obstructions

Breathe into your baby's mouth and nose

1 Open the airway and look, listen, and feel for breathing.

2 If your baby is not breathing, clear any visible obstruction from his mouth and nose.

3 Begin rescue breaths. Attempt FIVE initial rescue breaths into the mouth and nose. Go straight to step 4.

Give 30 chest compressions

Press down by one-third of the depth of the chest

4 Immediately give 30 chest compressions (this may dislodge obstruction), and TWO rescue breaths. Give 30 compressions to two rescue breaths for 1 minute.

☎ **CALL AN AMBULANCE**

Give 30 chest compressions

Follow with two breaths

5 Continue cycle of 30 chest compressions followed by two rescue breaths until help arrives, your baby resumes breathing, or you become too exhausted to continue.

» *see also*
● Unconscious baby, *pp.17–21*

Choking child

Start by asking your child if she is choking. If the blockage is mild, she will be able to speak, cough, and breathe. If it is severe, she will not be able to speak, cough, or breathe.

Give five back blows with heel of hand

Support child with other hand

Place a fist against the upper abdomen below the rib cage

Give five abdominal thrusts

1 If your child can cough, encourage her to do so to remove the object.

2 If your child can't talk, cough, or breathe, help her to bend forwards. Give her five sharp blows between the shoulder blades with the heel of your hand. Check her mouth. Remove any object you can see.

3 If the back blows fail, give abdominal thrusts. Place one fist in the middle of her upper abdomen, just below her rib cage. Cover your fist with your other hand. Give five upwards thrusts. Check your child's mouth.

4 If the abdominal thrusts fail, repeat steps 2 and 3 three times. If this is unsuccessful,

☎ **CALL AN AMBULANCE**

5 Continue cycles of back blows and abdominal thrusts until help arrives, the obstruction clears, or the child loses consciousness.

If your child becomes unconscious

If your choking child loses conscious treat as here. If he starts breathing at any stage, place him in the recovery position and SEEK MEDICAL ADVICE.

The recovery position

If the child starts breathing again but remains unconscious, place him in the recovery position and CALL AN AMBULANCE

Tilt head to open airway

1 Open his airway. Look, listen, and feel for breathing. If your child is not breathing, clear any visible obstruction from his mouth. Don't do a blind finger sweep.

Give five rescue breaths

2 Begin rescue breaths. Attempt FIVE initial rescue breaths into the mouth and nose. Go straight to step 3.

Place one hand on centre of the chest

Give 30 chest compressions

3 Immediately give 30 chest compressions (this may dislodge obstruction), then repeat TWO rescue breaths. Continue to give 30 compressions followed by two rescue breaths for 1 minute.

☎ **CALL AN AMBULANCE**

Give 30 chest compressions

4 Continue cycle of 30 chest compressions followed by two rescue breaths until help arrives, your child resumes breathing, or you become too exhausted to continue.

» see also
● Unconscious child, *pp.22–29*

Breath holding

This is the result of rage and frustration and it only happens in children under four years of age. Your child is breath holding if he cries, then breathes in but does not breathe out. He may go blue in the face and stiff and may even become unconscious momentarily.

Blow into his face

1 Try to stay calm. Do not shake him or make a fuss. He will usually start breathing again spontaneously.

2 Try blowing directly into his face; this often results in a child starting to breathe again.

» *see also*

● Unconscious child, *pp.22–29*

Hiccups

These are very common and usually only last for a few minutes, though often seems to go on for a long time. Children can become distressed.

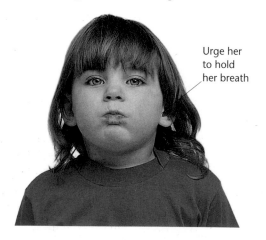

Urge her to hold her breath

1 Tell your child to sit still and to hold her breath for as long as she can. Then encourage her to breathe out slowly.

2 Get her to repeat this until hiccups have stopped.

Suffocation and strangulation

Strangulation results from a constriction around the child's neck that prevents breathing. Suffocation occurs when there is an obstruction over the mouth or nose, a weight on the child's chest or abdomen preventing normal breathing, or because the child is inhaling smoke- or fume-filled air, which prevents oxygen entering the lungs.

Remove constriction quickly

Look for chest movements

☎ CALL AN AMBULANCE

1 Remove the obstruction quickly. Use scissors to cut constriction if necessary. Breathing may restart.

2 Open your child's airway and check his breathing. If he is breathing, place him in the recovery position.

! IMPORTANT

● **If** your child is hanging, support his body while you remove or cut the rope or cord.

● **If** your child is not breathing, begin rescue breaths and chest compressions.

» see also

● Unconscious baby, *pp.17–21*

● Unconscious child, *pp.22–29*

Fume inhalation

Fume, gas, and smoke inhalation requires urgent medical attention as the fumes prevent the child breathing in oxygen.

Look for chest movements

Move your child into fresh air

☎ CALL AN AMBULANCE

1 Carry your child away from danger area. Ensure that you do not put yourself at risk.

2 Open her airway and check her breathing. If breathing, place her in the recovery position, and treat any injuries found.

! IMPORTANT

● **Do not** enter the area if fumes, gas, or smoke are still present. CALL FIRE SERVICE and AMBULANCE.

● **If** your child is not breathing, begin rescue breaths and chest compressions.

» see also

● Burns and scalds, *p.58*

● Unconscious baby, *pp.17–21*

● Unconscious child, *pp.22–29*

Croup

This condition can be alarming and usually occurs at night, but passes quickly. Your child will have: difficulty breathing, particularly *inhaling* and a short, barking cough. He may be making a crowing or whistling noise. In a severe attack, he may use muscles around his nose, neck, and upper arms in his attempts to breathe and he may have blue-tinged skin.

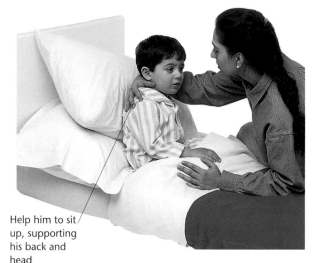

Help him to sit up, supporting his back and head

1 Help your child to sit up in bed. Prop him up with pillows at his back and head and reassure him.

Steam can ease his breathing

Keep your child well clear of hot running water

2 Create a steamy atmosphere; run hot water into the bath or boil a kettle in an enclosed room. Try to get your child to relax enough to breathe in the steam.

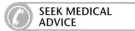 **SEEK MEDICAL ADVICE**

Asthma

If your child suffers from asthma, familiarise her with her medication so that she knows how to use it in an attack. You can recognise an attack if your child: has difficulty breathing and is coughing; is wheezing especially when breathing *out;* is distressed and anxious. She may also be tired by efforts to breathe and have a bluish tinge to face and lips.

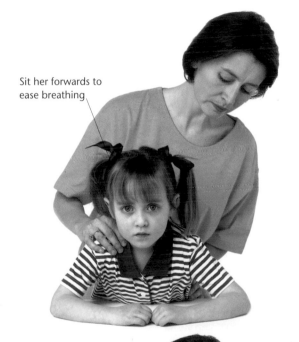

Sit her forwards to ease breathing

1 Ensure the room is well ventilated and smoke-free. If she has medication help her to use it, see right.

2 Help your child to relax. Sit her down in a comfortable breathing position with her arms resting on a table. Tell her to try to breathe slowly and deeply.

OR

3 If she is still uncomfortable, sit her on your lap, leaning slighty forwards. Reassure her as she will be frightened.

If she prefers, sit her on your lap

> **! IMPORTANT**
>
> • **If** it is a first attack, CALL AN AMBULANCE.
>
> • **If** the attack is severe, or does not respond to medication within 5 minutes, CALL AN AMBULANCE.
>
> • **If** your child has special medication, use it early in any attack.

Using medication

If your child has medication, let him use it. Make sure you give him the reliever inhaler – this normally has a blue cap. (Preventer inhalers have brown or white caps.) For best results, especially with children, inhalers are fitted with plastic "spacers"; follow the directions carefully. The attack should ease within 3 minutes. If it doesn't, repeat dose.

Bleeding

Severe bleeding can be distressing for you and your child. If it is not controlled your child may develop a life-threatening condition known as shock. Large wounds may need stitches.

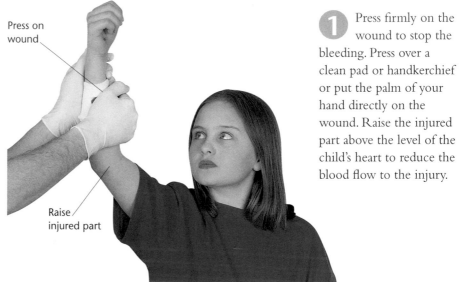

Press on wound

Raise injured part

1 Press firmly on the wound to stop the bleeding. Press over a clean pad or handkerchief or put the palm of your hand directly on the wound. Raise the injured part above the level of the child's heart to reduce the blood flow to the injury.

Lay child down, keeping injured part high

Keep pressing on wound

2 Help your child to lie down, with her head low (you can put a thin pad under her head for comfort). Keep the injured part raised above her heart. Continue to press on the wound for up to 10 minutes.

Keep her head low – use a thin pad for comfort

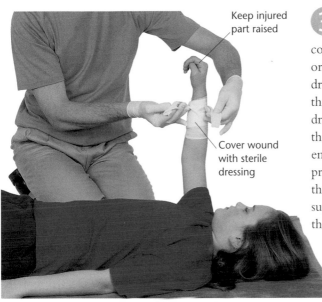

Keep injured part raised

Cover wound with sterile dressing

3 Keeping the injured part raised, cover the wound and original pad with a sterile dressing that is larger than the wound. Secure the dressing with a bandage; the bandage must be firm enough to maintain pressure, but not so tight that it cuts off the blood supply to the area beyond the injury.

When bleeding stops

Once the bleeding is under control, or stops, support the injury in a raised position – for example, with an elevation sling, *see p.107.* TAKE YOUR CHILD TO HOSPITAL.

Keep injured part raised

Raise legs above her heart

4 If bleeding is still not under control, keep injury high but in addition, raise her legs higher than her chest and support them on cushions. Remove the pad from under her head. Loosen any tight clothing and, if necessary, cover her with a blanket to keep her warm. If she is thirsty, moisten her lips with water, but don't let her drink or eat.

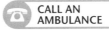 **CALL AN AMBULANCE**

Lower head

>> *see also*
- Embedded object, *p.46*
- Shock, *p.30*

Embedded object

A large object such as a piece of glass that becomes stuck in a wound is serious as it may be plugging the wound, preventing bleeding. Protect it with padding and bandages and get your child to medical help.

Bandaging around larger objects

If the object is very big, build up padding around it, then bandage above and below the object instead of over the top.

Raise injured part above his heart

Press either side of the wound

1 Help your child to lie down and keep him calm. Apply pressure on either side of the object, pushing the edges together. Raise the injured part above the level of your child's heart.

Drape a piece of gauze over wound

Place padding around the object

2 Place a piece of gauze over the wound and object to minimise the risk of infection. Build up padding to the same height as the embedded object; spare bandages are ideal for this.

3 Secure padding by bandaging over it, being careful not to press on the embedded object.

Bandage over padding and object

see also
● Bleeding, p.44

☎ **CALL AN AMBULANCE**

OR

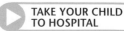
▶ **TAKE YOUR CHILD TO HOSPITAL**

Cuts and grazes

Children can be very upset by the tiniest graze. Ressure your child and wash the wound. Covering the wound with a plaster keeps it clean and often makes the child feel better.

Sit child down

Wash graze

1 Help your child to sit down and reassure her. Gently wash the graze with soap and water using a gauze pad or a very soft brush. If the wound is very dirty rinse under cold running water.

Remove any loose dirt

2 Try to remove any loose particles of dirt or gravel. This may cause slight bleeding.

Press clean pad on graze

3 Apply pressure with a clean pad to stop any bleeding. Pat the wound dry with clean pieces of gauze.

Protect graze with a plaster

4 Cover the cut or graze with a plaster that has a pad large enough to cover the wound and the area around it.

》 see also
● Infected wound, *p.48*

! **IMPORTANT**

● **Do not** try to remove objects that are embedded in a wound as you may cause further damage and bleeding.

Tetanus

This is a dangerous infection that is present in the soil. If it is transferred into a wound, tetanus germs release toxins (poisons) into the nervous system. Tetanus is best prevented through vaccination. Babies receive this as part of their immunisation programme. Every child should be given a tetanus booster before starting school.

Infected wound

A wound is infected if there is: increasing pain and soreness; swelling, redness, and a feeling of heat around the injury; pus within, or oozing from, the wound; swelling and tenderness in the glands in the neck, armpit, or groin; and possible faint red trails on the skin leading to these glands. When infection is advanced there may also be signs of fever (sweating, thirst, shivering, and lethargy).

Cover wound with a clean pad

Bandage dressing in place

1 Cover the wound with a clean non-fluffy pad or sterile dressing secured in place with a bandage.

2 Raise the infected wound, and support it, for example, with an elevation sling.

SEEK MEDICAL ADVICE

Raise and support injury

» **see also**

● Triangular bandages, p.106

Blisters

If a blister is caused by friction (for example, a badly fitting shoe) treat as here. You can get special padded blister plasters to keep in a first aid kit.

! IMPORTANT

● **If** the blister is very large, cover it with a clean, non-fluffy dressing, held in place with adhesive tape or a bandage.

● **Never** deliberately break a blister as this can cause it to become infected.

● **Do not** use this method for a blister caused by a burn.

Clean blister with soap and water

1 Clean the blister thoroughly with soap and water. Rinse it with clean water.

Pat dry with clean pad

2 Thoroughly dry the blister and the surrounding skin. Pat it gently with a clean gauze pad or paper tissues.

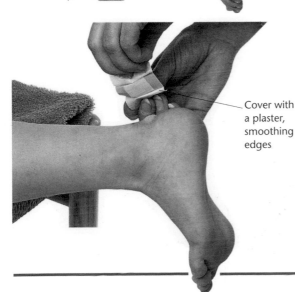

Cover with a plaster, smoothing edges

3 Cover the blister with an ordinary plaster, or blister plaster if you have one. Make sure the edges are smooth, to prevent another blister developing. The plaster needs to have a pad large enough to cover the entire blister.

» see also

● Burns and scalds, *p.58*

! IMPORTANT

● **Do not** try to remove objects in the eye.

● **If** you cannot transport your child lying on his back, CALL AN AMBULANCE.

Eye wound

This type of wound is serious because of the risk of damage to the child's sight. Injury can scar the surface of the eye or lead to infection.

Tell him to keep both eyes still

Lay the child down

Keep his head supported

1 Help your child to lie down down and cradle his head in your lap to keep it still. He may be in pain, tell him not to rub or move either of his eyes. If he moves his good eye, the injured one will move too, which may damage it even more.

Cover injured eye with a sterile dressing

2 Reassure your child and then cover the injured eye with a sterile dressing. Hold the dressing in place until you get medical help.

3 Keep him lying on his back.

▶ **TAKE YOUR CHILD TO HOSPITAL**

⟫ see also

● Chemical burn to eye, *p.62*

● Object in eye, *p.82*

Nosebleed

Children get nosebleeds from a blow to the nose, or from picking it. Bleeding usually stops quickly, but it can alarm young children.

Tilt her head forwards

Pinch the soft part of the nose below the bone

1 Help your child to sit down with her head well forwards. Ask her to breathe through her mouth, then pinch the fleshy part of her nose for 10 minutes. Then release the pressure.

Keep her head forwards

Pinch for further 10 minutes if bleeding has not stopped

Let her dribble or spit into a bowl

2 Tell your child to spit out any excess fluid in her mouth. If the bleeding has not stopped, pinch again for another 10 minutes, then release pressure. If the nose is still bleeding, pinch again.

Tell her not to blow her nose

Clean with warm water

3 Once the bleeding has stopped, use some cotton wool dipped in lukewarm water to clean your child's face. Advise her to rest and not to blow her nose. If your child picks at (or blows) her nose within the next few hours, the bleeding may start again.

» see also
● Head injury, *p.66*

! IMPORTANT

● **If** the bleeding follows a head injury and there is thin, watery fluid draining from the ear, CALL AN AMBULANCE.

● **If** the injury is caused by an earring being ripped out, your child may need stitches. TAKE YOUR CHILD TO HOSPITAL.

Bleeding from inside the ear

Help your child into a semi-upright position, with his head tilted towards the injured side, to allow blood to drain away. Put an absorbent pad over the ear and bandage it lightly in place. Do not plug the ear. SEEK MEDICAL ADVICE.

≫ *see also*

● Object in ear, *p.83*
● Head injury, *p.66*

Ear wound

Outer ear wounds can bleed profusely, which can be alarming. If blood is coming from inside the ear, check that your child has not inserted something into it. If bleeding follows a head injury, call an ambulance.

Press on wound over a clean pad for 10 minutes

1 Help your child to sit down and gently pinch the wound with your thumb and forefinger over a clean piece of gauze. Keep pressing for 10 minutes.

Bandage to keep wound covered

2 Cover the injured ear with a sterile dressing and lightly bandage it in place.

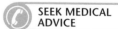

SEEK MEDICAL ADVICE

Mouth wound

These wounds can be the result of a child biting the inside of his mouth in a fall, for example, or from the loss of a tooth. Make sure your child does not inhale blood, as this can result in breathing problems.

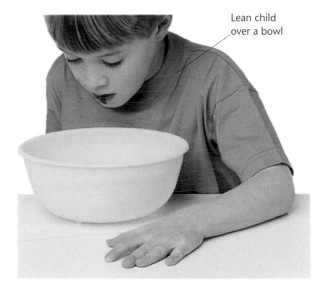

Lean child over a bowl

1 Help your child to sit down with his head over a bowl. Encourage him to spit out any blood.

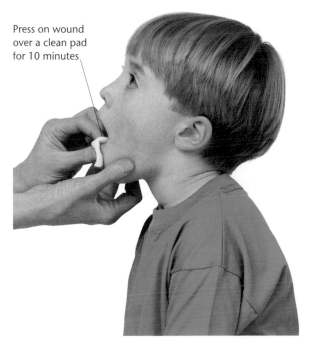

Press on wound over a clean pad for 10 minutes

2 Place a pad over the wound and pinch it between your thumb and forefinger, maintaining the pressure for 10 minutes. Your child may be able to do this for himself.

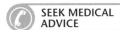
SEEK MEDICAL ADVICE

! IMPORTANT

● **Do not** wash out his mouth as this may disturb a blood clot.

● **If** he loses a tooth, it may be possible to replant an "adult" tooth. Do not clean the tooth; put it in milk. TAKE YOUR CHILD TO THE DENTIST.

● **Ensure** a milk tooth has not been inhaled or swallowed. A dentist should check the gum.

Bleeding from tooth socket

Place a pad over the tooth socket, making sure that it is higher than the adjacent teeth so that your child can bite on it. Ask your child to sit down with her hand supporting her jaw. Tell her to bite hard on the pad. A younger child may need you to hold the pad in place.

Care of the amputated part

Wrap the severed part in kitchen film or a plastic bag. Wrap the bag in a soft fabric, such as a cotton handkerchief or piece of gauze. Put a plastic bag filled with ice cubes around the fabric. This helps preserve the severed part until you get to hospital. Put the whole package in another bag or container. Mark with the time of injury and the child's name and give it to the ambulance personnel.

Amputation

Whether a injury causes partial or total amputation, the limb can often be reattached. Your child will need an anaesthetic so don't give him anything to eat or drink because it will delay surgery.

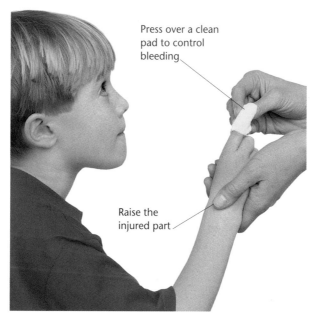

Press over a clean pad to control bleeding

Raise the injured part

1 Control the blood loss by pressing firmly on the injury using a sterile dressing or clean pad. Raise the injured part above the level of your child's heart. If necessary, help your child to lie down and raise his legs above his heart.

2 Bandage or tape the dressing firmly in place. You can cover a finger with a gauze finger bandage to protect it.

📞 CALL AN AMBULANCE

Bandage the pad

3 Tell the ambulance control it is an amputation. Monitor your child for signs of shock while waiting. If possible, put the severed part in a plastic bag, see left.

» *see also*
● Bleeding, *p.44*
● Shock, *p.30*

Internal bleeding

Suspect this when signs of shock develop without obvious blood loss. There may also be "pattern bruising" around the injury with marks from clothes or crushing objects. There could also be bleeding from orifices, such as the nose or ear. Note what this looks like and keep a sample.

Raise and support her legs

Cover her with a blanket

Keep her head low

 CALL AN AMBULANCE

1 Help her to lie down; raise her legs.

2 Monitor breathing and pulse rate while waiting for help.

> **! IMPORTANT**
>
> ● **If** child is unconscious, open her airway and check breathing. If breathing, place in the recovery position; if not breathing, begin rescue breaths and chest compressions.

> **» see also**
>
> ● Shock, *p.30*
> ● Unconscious baby, *pp.17–21*
> ● Unconscious child, *pp.22–29*

Crush injury

A crush injury can be serious as it may cause internal bleeding and broken bones as well as open wounds.

Remove the object quickly

Press on wound to control bleeding

 CALL AN AMBULANCE

1 If the accident has only just happened, remove the heavy object from the child quickly.

2 Control any bleeding by pressing firmly on the wound, with your hand or a clean pad. Support the injured part but do not move it.

> **! IMPORTANT**
>
> ● **If** your child has been crushed for more than 15 minutes, do not remove the object as this increases the risk of shock and further internal injury.
>
> ● **If** you suspect broken bones, support the injury but do not move your child unless he is in immediate danger. Watch for signs of shock while waiting for the ambulance.

> **» see also**
>
> ● Bleeding, *p.44*
> ● Shock, *p.30*

IMPORTANT

- **Monitor** your child for signs of shock.

- **If** child loses consciousness, open his airway and check breathing. If breathing, place in the recovery position; if not breathing, begin rescue breaths and chest compressions.

Chest wound

A chest wound may cause severe internal injuries. The lungs are particularly vulnerable, and breathing problems, shock, and collapsed lungs may follow an injury. It is important to make an airtight seal over the wound to prevent air entering the chest cavity.

Support him in semi-upright position

Cover wound with your hand

1 Cover the wound with the palm of your hand and support your child in a semi-upright position. Reassure your child.

Place clean pad over wound

Cover pad with kitchen film and tape three sides

2 With your child supported, cover the wound with a sterile dressing or clean pad and tape it in place on three sides, *far left*. Cover the pad with kitchen film to seal it; again secure tape on only three sides, *left*.

3 Incline your child towards his injured side, supported with cushions. This helps support his chest.

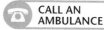

CALL AN AMBULANCE

Turn child to lean on injured side

see also

- Bleeding, *p.44*
- Shock, *p.30*
- Unconscious child, *pp.22–29*

Abdominal injury

A child with an abdominal injury is likely to develop the signs of shock. There is high risk of internal as well as external bleeding.

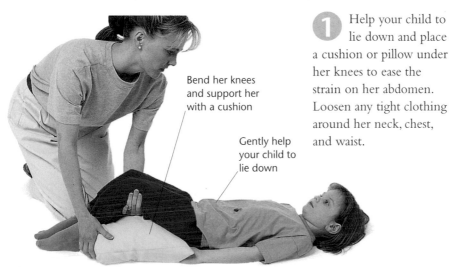

Bend her knees and support her with a cushion

Gently help your child to lie down

1 Help your child to lie down and place a cushion or pillow under her knees to ease the strain on her abdomen. Loosen any tight clothing around her neck, chest, and waist.

Cover wound with dressing

2 Reassure your child while you place a large sterile dressing over the wound. Support the wound with your hand if your child wants to cough or is going to vomit.

Tape dressing in place

3 Use adhesive tape to secure the dressing lightly in place.

☎ CALL AN AMBULANCE

4 Continue to reassure her and watch for any change in her condition while waiting for help.

» see also
● Bleeding, *p.44*
● Shock, *p.30*
● Unconscious child, *pp.22–29*

- **Do not** remove any clothing or material that may be sticking to the burned area as this may cause further damage to the skin.

- **If** no cold water is available, use another cool liquid such as milk.

- **Do not** immerse young children in cold water as this can cause hypothermia.

- **Do not** touch the burn or burst any blisters.

Burns to the mouth and throat

Burns in this area are very serious as they cause swelling and inflammation of the air passages, giving a serious risk of suffocation. Act quickly. If necessary, loosen clothing from around her neck. If your child develops breathing difficulties, open her airway and check breathing. If she is not breathing begin rescue breaths and chest compressions. CALL AN AMBULANCE.

Burns and scalds

You must seek medical advice for all burns on children. A child with a large burn must be taken to hospital. It is very important to cool the burn as quickly as possible to minimise damage.

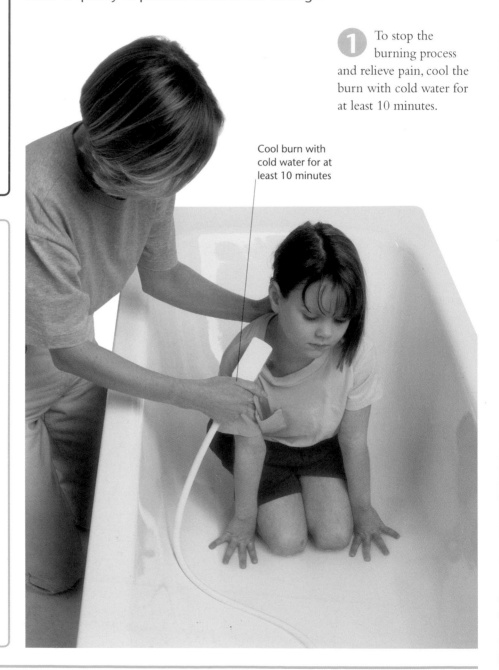

1 To stop the burning process and relieve pain, cool the burn with cold water for at least 10 minutes.

Cool burn with cold water for at least 10 minutes

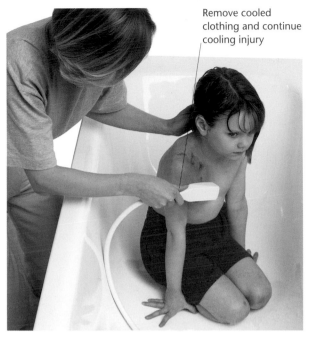

Remove cooled clothing and continue cooling injury

2 Once cooled, remove clothing from the burned area and, if the pain persists, cool again. Cut around any material that is sticking to the skin. Remove jewellery and all restrictive clothing from around the burn (for example, belts or watches) before any swelling occurs.

! IMPORTANT

● **Never** put lotions, fat, or ointment on a burn or scald.

● **If** the burn covers a large part of the child, CALL AN AMBULANCE.

● **Do not** give your child anything to eat or drink and watch for signs of shock.

● **If** child loses consciousness, open airway and check breathing. If breathing, place in the recovery position; if not breathing, begin rescue breaths and chest compressions. CALL AN AMBULANCE.

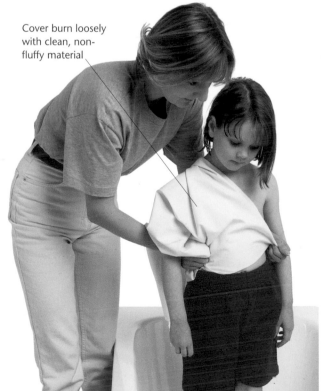

Cover burn loosely with clean, non-fluffy material

3 Cover the burn with clean, non-fluffy material to protect it from infection. You can use a clean sheet or pillow case. The dressing does not need to be secured. Ensure that your child remains warm to prevent the onset of hypothermia.

▶ **TAKE YOUR CHILD TO HOSPITAL**

» *see also*
● Fire, *p.11*
● Shock, *p.30*
● Unconscious baby, *pp.17–21*
● Unconscious child, *pp.22–29*

Alternative dressings

To protect a burned hand or foot you can use a plastic bag or clean kitchen film, both of which will protect the burn from infection. Secure the bag with a bandage or plaster around the bag, not the skin.

Electrical burn test

An electric shock from a low-voltage source can result in burns. These may occur at both the point of entry and the point of exit of the current.

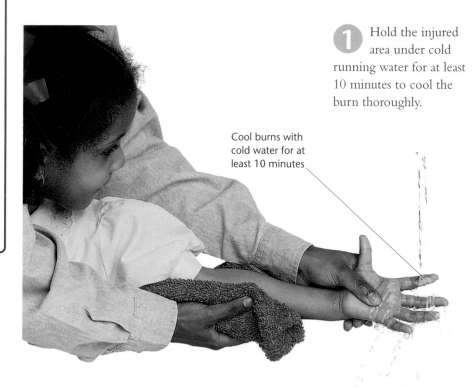

1 Hold the injured area under cold running water for at least 10 minutes to cool the burn thoroughly.

Cool burns with cold water for at least 10 minutes

Cover burns with clean plastic bag

2 Protect the burn by covering it with clean, non–fluffy material or with a plastic bag, held or taped in place.

▶ **TAKE YOUR CHILD TO HOSPITAL**

⟫ see also

● Electrical injury, *p.12*

● Unconscious baby, *pp.17–21*

● Unconscious child, *p.22–29*

Chemical burn to skin

Chemical burns can be caused by household agents such as oven cleaner or paint stripper. These burns are serious and there will be: fierce, stinging pain; redness or staining, followed by blistering and peeling of skin.

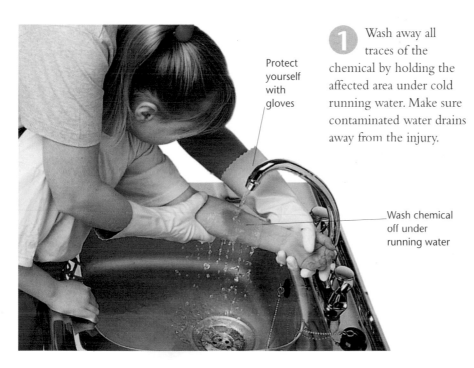

Protect yourself with gloves

Wash chemical off under running water

1 Wash away all traces of the chemical by holding the affected area under cold running water. Make sure contaminated water drains away from the injury.

Cover burn loosely with clean, non-fluffy material

2 Loosely cover the burn with clean, non-fluffy material, such as a pillow case. This avoids constriction when the wound swells. You can wet the pillow case to cool and soothe the burn.

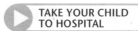
TAKE YOUR CHILD TO HOSPITAL

! IMPORTANT

● **Note** the name of the substance that caused the burn and give the information to the hospital staff.

● **Always** wear protective gloves when treating your child, and beware of chemical fumes.

Removing clothes

Cut clothing away from the affected area, unless you can slip it off without touching other parts of the body. Avoid cutting through the affected clothing – cut around it instead.

» *see also*

● Chemical burn to eye, *p.62*

● Fume inhalation, *p.41*

● Swallowed chemicals, *p.63*

! IMPORTANT

● **Do not** let your child touch his eye. The eye will be shut in spasm and pain, so gently pull the eyelids open.

Chemical burn to eye

Splashes of chemicals in the eye can cause scarring or even blindness. Your child may have a chemical burn if he complains of fierce pain in the eye; he has difficulty opening the affected eye; the surface of the eye is watery; there is redness and swelling in and around the eye.

Using a jug of water

If you can't hold your child under a tap, and you have help, you may find it easier to use a jug to pour water over the affected eye. Get the helper to support the child with her head tilted down and to one side. Avoid splashing the "good" eye with the contaminated water.

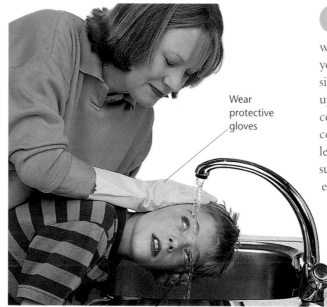

Wear protective gloves

Rinse eye with cold water for 10 minutes

1 Protect yourself from the chemical with rubber gloves. Hold your child's head over a sink, with the "good" eye uppermost. Gently run cold water over the contaminated eye for at least 10 minutes. Make sure that both sides of the eyelid are thoroughly washed and that the contaminated water drains away from your child's face.

Cover eye with clean pad

2 Once the injured eye is thoroughly washed, cover it with a large sterile dressing. Hold the dressing in place until you get medical aid.

CALL AN AMBULANCE

OR

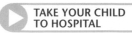
TAKE YOUR CHILD TO HOSPITAL

Swallowed chemicals

If you think your child has swallowed a poison, try to find out how much. Be aware too that some chemicals also give off dangerous fumes.

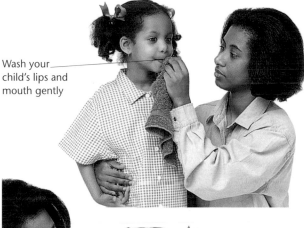

Wash your child's lips and mouth gently

 IMPORTANT
- **Do not** try to make your child vomit as this can cause further harm.

- **If** your child loses consciousness, open her airway and check breathing. If breathing, place her in the recovery position; if not breathing, begin rescue breaths and chest compressions.

1 Wipe away any residual chemical from around your child's mouth and face.

Help her take sips of cold water or milk

2 Her lips may be burned or discoloured, so give her frequent sips of cold water or milk to cool the lips.

 CALL AN AMBULANCE

Keep container to show medical team

3 Find out what chemical your child swallowed and if possible how much, then tell the emergency services when you make the call. This will help them determine the correct treatment.

>> *see also*
- Chemical burn to eye, *p.62*
- Fume inhalation, *p.41*
- Unconscious baby, *pp.17–21*
- Unconscious child, *pp.22–29*

›› see also

● Unconscious baby, *pp.17–21*

● Unconscious child, *p.22–29*

Drug or alcohol poisoning

If your child has taken medication the container may be nearby. If he drank alcohol there may be a smell of alcohol and he may be staggering and be sick. He may also have: a flushed and moist face; slurred speech; deep noisy breathing; a bounding pulse.

Keep container

Count how many pills are left

1 If your child is conscious, try to find out what he has taken and how much. Check the label on the medicine bottle and tell ambulance control when you ring.

☎ CALL AN AMBULANCE

2 If he drank alcohol, let your child rest where you can watch him while waiting for the ambulance. Give him a bowl in case he is sick. If he falls asleep, try to wake him to make sure he can be easily roused.

Plant poisoning

Many plants are poisonous in large quantities. Small pieces or one or two berries are unlikely to be fatal but can cause stomach upset.

Check his mouth and tell him to spit out any pieces

1 Try to find out what your child has eaten and keep a sample to show the doctor.

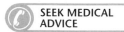
☎ SEEK MEDICAL ADVICE

2 Look inside your child's mouth. Pick out any remaining pieces of plant or berries.

Scalp wound

This type of wound can bleed profusely. If the wound was caused by a blow to the child's head, watch for any change in her condition, especially her level of consciousness, while waiting for the ambulance.

Place a pad on wound

Apply firm, steady pressure

1 Cover the injury with a clean pad or sterile dressing that is larger than the wound. Press firmly on the pad and the wound to control the bleeding. Place another pad on top, if necessary, and keep pressing on the wound.

Secure bandage firmly but not too tightly

2 Bandage the dressing firmly in place. If the bleeding continues, apply pressure again with your hand.

Keep her head and shoulders slightly raised

Help her to lie down

3 Help your child to lie down with her head and shoulders slightly raised. Watch for any changes in her condition.

☎ **CALL AN AMBULANCE**

> **! IMPORTANT**
>
> ● **If** blood continues to seep through the two dressings, remove both pads and apply a new dressing.
>
> ● **If** your child loses consciousness, open her airway and check breathing. If breathing, place in the recovery position; if not breathing, begin rescue breaths and chest compressions.

》 *see also*

● Bleeding, *p.44*

● Head injury, *p.66*

● Unconscious baby, *pp.17–21*

● Unconscious child, *pp.22–29*

Skull fracture

Fractures of the skull are very serious injuries. Skull fracture can result in bleeding within the brain, which causes compression. Suspect skull fracture if there is: a wound on your child's head; a soft area on the scalp; consciousness is impaired; clear fluid coming from the nose or ear; blood showing on the white of the eye; or, distortion of the face or head. CALL AN AMBULANCE.

Head injury

If your child has a minor bump on the head, he may simply have a small bruise with no other sign of injury. With concussion the child's brain is "shaken" by the blow; he may be dazed or temporarily unconscious (about 20 seconds), but recovers completely. He may have a headache, feel dizzy, complain of nausea, and may not remember what happened.

In compression, blood accumulates within the skull, pressing on the brain. The child may seem unaffected at first, however, hours (or days) later he deteriorates. He may be disorientated, drowsy, and confused. He may have: a severe headache; a fever; weakness or paralysis down one side; and unequal pupils. Eventually he will be unconscious with a strong, slow pulse, and noisy breathing that becomes very slow.

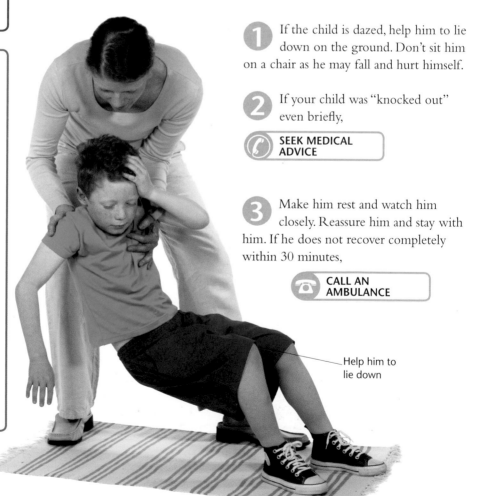

1 If the child is dazed, help him to lie down on the ground. Don't sit him on a chair as he may fall and hurt himself.

2 If your child was "knocked out" even briefly,

✆ **SEEK MEDICAL ADVICE**

3 Make him rest and watch him closely. Reassure him and stay with him. If he does not recover completely within 30 minutes,

☎ **CALL AN AMBULANCE**

Help him to lie down

Checking a child's level of consciousness

Your child could be awake following an injury, fully unconscious and not respond to you at all, or somewhere between the two. He may deteriorate. It is important to assess his condition and monitor any changes so that you can tell the ambulance personnel or hospital staff.

- Is he alert? Does he respond normally when you talk to him?

- Does he answer simple questions or obey instructions?

- Is he completely unresponsive?

Note down any response, or change in response (with the time of the change).

Put compress on injury and monitor condition

If your child loses consciousness

Do not move your child as there could be an associated back or neck injury and moving her could result in damage to the brain or spinal cord.

Lift jaw to open airway

1 Kneel behind her head and open her airway using the jaw thrust as follows. Place one hand on either side of her face, with your fingertips on the angles of her jaw. Gently lift the jaw to open the airway (don't tilt her head back).

Check breathing

2 Check her breathing. If she is breathing, leave her as she is and continue to support her jaw to keep the airway open. If she is not breathing, begin rescue breaths and chest compressions.

 CALL AN AMBULANCE

 see also
- Cold compresses, *p.108*
- Spine injury, *pp.69–71*
- Scalp wound, *p.65*
- Unconscious baby, *pp.17–21*
- Unconscious child, *pp.22–29*

! IMPORTANT

- **If** pinching her nose hurts too much, simply ask her to sit forward over the bowl and give her a soft pad or towel to soak up the blood.

Nose/cheekbone injury

The main risk with injuries to the nose or cheek is that the swelling can affect the air passages causing breathing problems. There may also be bleeding from the child's nose or mouth.

Apply cold compress to injury

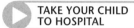

Pinch nostrils together to stop bleeding

≫ see also

- Nosebleed, *p.51*
- Unconscious baby, *pp.17–21*
- Unconscious child, *pp.22–29*

1 Help your child to sit down and apply a cold compress to the injured area. This helps to reduce the swelling. Hold the compress in place for about 30 minutes.

2 If your child's nose is bleeding heavily, ask her to sit with her head over a bowl and to pinch her nostrils together to help control it.

▶ **TAKE YOUR CHILD TO HOSPITAL**

! IMPORTANT

- **If** your child loses consciousness, open airway and check her breathing. If not breathing, begin rescue breaths and chest compressions. CALL AN AMBULANCE.

Jaw injury

If your child has a broken jaw it will be tender, swollen, and bruised. Her teeth may be out of line.

Hold pad against jaw and support jaw with your hand

≫ see also

- Unconscious baby, *pp.17–21*
- Unconscious child, *p.22–29*

1 Help your child to sit down with head well forwards. Tell her not to swallow but to let any blood or saliva drain away.

2 Make a soft pad and hold it firmly under her injured jaw. Do not bandage the pad in place in case she is sick. Continue to support the jaw on the way to the hospital.

▶ **TAKE YOUR CHILD TO HOSPITAL**

Spine injury

If a child lands on his neck or back in a fall or fell awkwardly and complains of back pain or tingling in any part of his body, suspect spine injury. Support him in the position you found him to minimise damage.

⚠ IMPORTANT

● **Do not** move the injured child unless his life is in danger.

● **If** you do have to move him, try to do so in "one piece", taking care not to twist or bend the neck or spine.

Support his head in your hands

Leave a slight gap so that your child can hear you

Keep his back straight

1 Reassure your child and tell him not to move. Steady and support his head and neck by placing your hands over his ears and keeping his head in line with his spine. Be careful not to pull on his neck.

☎ **CALL AN AMBULANCE**

Continue to support his head

Place rolled blankets around his head and shoulders

2 Keep his head supported in this position until help arrives. Ask someone to put rolled blankets or towels around his neck and shoulders for extra support.

Place folded blankets or towels either side of his body

3 Ask your helper to arrange rolled towels or blankets along either side of his body while you continue to keep his head steady.

≫ see also

● Spine injury if unconscious, *p.70*

● Unconscious baby, *pp.17–21*

● Unconscious child, *p.22–29*

Spine injury if unconscious

If your child is unconscious following a fall on to his back, you should follow the usual steps to treat unconsciousness, but you need to adapt how you open his airway to prevent movement of the back or neck.

Tap his shoulder

Keep head and body aligned

CALL AN AMBULANCE

1 Keep your child's head, trunk, and toes in a straight line. Check for a response by tapping his shoulder.

Place your fingertips at the angle of the jaw

2 Open his airway using the jaw thrust. Kneel behind his head and place your hands on either side of his face, with your fingertips at the angles of his jaw. Gently lift his jaw to open the airway; make sure you don't tilt his head.

Feel for breathing

3 Check his breathing. If he is not breathing begin rescue breaths and chest compressions. If he is breathing, support his head until help arrives. If you can't maintain an open airway, place him in the recovery position (*see opposite* and *p.28*).

» see also

● Unconscious baby, *pp.17–21*

● Unconscious child, *p.22–29*

If you have one helper

If your child is breathing and you can't maintain an open airway using the jaw lift, for example, if he vomits, place him in the recovery position.

1 Ask your helper to support your child's head with her hands. Grasp the thigh of the leg furthest from you. Gently lift and bend the leg. Bring furthest arm across the child's chest and place his hand against his face.

2 Holding the hand against his face, pull your child's knee towards you and ease him over gently. You and the helper should keep his head and trunk aligned at all times.

3 With your child on his side, maintain an open airway and support him in this position until help arrives. Monitor his breathing and pulse. If he stops breathing at any point begin rescue breaths and chest compressions without delay.

Lift and bend the leg

Get help to support head and neck

Straighten his leg very gently

Place back of hand against his cheek

Keep head supported

Draw over his knee

Ease child over

Keep head and neck supported

Bend uppermost leg to prevent him rolling forwards

For two or more helpers

If you have two or more adult helpers, use the "log-roll" technique to turn a child who is breathing. It is vital to keep his head, trunk, and feet in a straight line. While one adult holds the child's head, two others should gently straighten the limbs and roll the child over in one synchronised movement.

One helper supports arms and legs and pulls gently

Keep head in line with body while he is turned

One helper keeps trunk straight

Pelvic injury

If your child has a broken pelvis she will be unable to stand, with pain around the hip and groin, and possible bleeding from the urinary orifice.

Support leg at joints above and below injury

📞 **CALL AN AMBULANCE**

Place padding between child's legs. Immobilise them with a figure-of-eight bandage around feet and ankles, and a broad-fold bandage around both knees.

Leg injury

Suspect a break if your child is in severe pain. He needs an X-ray or scan to confirm whether or not a bone is broken. Keep him as still as possible to prevent broken bone ends causing further internal injury.

Support leg at joints above and below injury

1 Help your child to lie down gently and support his leg at both the ankle and knee joints. If possible ask someone to help you.

2 Place padding around the injured leg. Pad outside the injured limb and between the legs with rolled-up blankets. Cover your child with another blanket to keep him warm.

Make a J-shaped pad with a rolled blanket and place it around his leg

📞 **CALL AN AMBULANCE**

How to splint an injured leg

1 If the ambulance will be longer than 20 minutes, splint the injured leg. Gently pad between the thighs, knees, and ankles using rolled-up towels or small blankets. Carefully bring the uninjured leg alongside the broken limb.

Place plenty of soft padding between the legs

Support injured leg

2 Tie a narrow-fold figure-of-eight bandage around the feet and ankles to immobilise the leg.

Tie narrow-fold bandage in figure-of-eight at ankles and feet

3 Tie broad-fold bandages around the knee, and above as well as below the injury if there is room.

Tie reef knots on uninjured side

Tie broad-fold bandages at knees and above and below injury

Slide broad-fold under knee and tie ends together

Making broad-fold and narrow-fold bandages

1 Take a triangular bandage

2 Fold top point over to touch the base

3 Fold bandage in half to make a broad-fold bandage

BROAD-FOLD BANDAGE

4 Fold bandage in half again to make a narrow-fold bandage

NARROW-FOLD BANDAGE

! IMPORTANT

● **Do not** attempt to force the knee straight as this may cause further injury.

● **Do not** allow your child to walk on his injured leg.

● **Do not** give your child anything to eat or drink.

» see also

● Leg injury, *p.72*

Knee injury

This type of injury can be very painful, and your child may not be able to move it. The area around the knee joint can swell very quickly.

Support his knee with a pillow

Wrap padding around joint and bandage

Keep him comfortable

1 Help your child to lie down, then slide a pillow under his injured knee to provide support. Pad around the injured knee with cotton wool or a soft dressing, secured with a roller bandage.

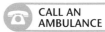
☎ CALL AN AMBULANCE

2 Reassure your child and keep him comfortable while you wait for the ambulance.

Foot injury

Your child's foot may be bruised, swollen, and stiff and she may not be able to stand. If caused by crushing, one or more bones may be broken.

Reduce swelling with an ice pack

Keep leg elevated

1 Help your child to sit down. Raise and support her injured foot.

2 Place a cold compress against the injury to relieve pain and minimise swelling (*see p.108*). Secure compress in place with a bandage.

» see also

● Leg injury, *p.72*

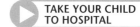
▶ TAKE YOUR CHILD TO HOSPITAL

Ankle injury

The most common injury is a sprain. Suspect a sprain if your child can't take her full weight on her foot after a fall, or she has twisted, or wrenched, her ankle. She may need an X-ray or scan.

IMPORTANT

● **If** the pain is very severe or you think a bone could be broken, treat as for a leg injury and TAKE YOUR CHILD TO HOSPITAL or CALL AN AMBULANCE.

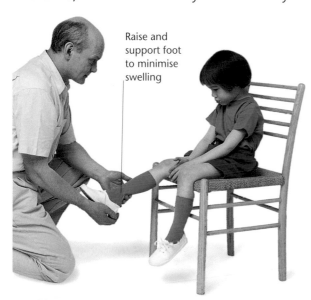

Raise and support foot to minimise swelling

1 Help your child to sit down to rest her foot. Raise her foot and gently remove her sock and shoe before the injured area swells.

Apply a cold compress

2 To minimise swelling, place a cold compress on the injury. Use a flannel wrung out in cold water or an icepack (*see p.108*).

Secure padding with a bandage

Keep ankle raised and supported

3 Wrap the ankle with a thick layer of cotton wool. Bandage the cotton wool firmly in place. Support the ankle in a raised position.

see also

● Leg injury, *p.72*

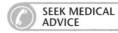

SEEK MEDICAL ADVICE

Collarbone injury

A collarbone may be broken by indirect force, for example, if a child falls onto his outstretched hand, or by a blow to his shoulder. There will be tenderness in your child's shoulder and arm – increased by attempts to move it – and his head will be turned and inclined to the injured side.

For additional support around a sling

A sling will support the arm on the injured side, but a broad-fold bandage provides extra support if you are taking your child to hospital by car. Make a broad-fold bandage (*see p.73*). Place some padding between the child's arm chest and tie the bandage right around the child's arm and chest. Tie the ends in a reef knot on his uninjured side.

>> *see also*
● Triangular bandages, p.106

Sit child down

Rest child's fingers on opposite shoulder

Place arm on injured side across his chest

1 Help your child to sit down and gently bring the arm on the injured side across his chest. Ask him to support his elbow with his hand.

Support arm with an elevation sling

Place padding between arm and body

2 Place your child's arm in an elevation sling for support and to minimse swelling and discomfort. Secure the sling with a reef knot.

Tie a broad-fold bandage around arm and body

3 Tie a broad-fold bandage around the arm and body for extra support.

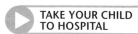
▶ TAKE YOUR CHILD TO HOSPITAL

Rib injury

A child may have a broken rib following a blow to his chest, a heavy fall, or having been crushed. Symptoms include: sharp pain at the fracture site; and pain on breathing. Suspect internal injury if you see signs of internal bleeding or an open wound.

Support child semi-upright, leaning towards injured side

Seal wound with pad and kitchen film taped in place

Raise arm on injured side across his chest

Put arm on injured side in elevation sling

 IMPORTANT

● **If** your child loses consciousness or develops breathing difficulties, open airway and check breathing. If breathing place him in the recovery position leaning on the injured side; if not breathing, begin rescue breaths and chest compressions.

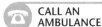 **CALL AN AMBULANCE**

1 If there is a wound, or several ribs injured support the chest wall to safeguard breathing. Support your child in a semi-upright position leaning towards his injured side. Seal any chest wound: place a sterile pad over the wound, cover this with kitchen film secured on three sides with tape.

2 Place the arm on the injured side across your child's chest for extra support.

3 Secure the raised arm in an elevation sling. Keep him as comfortable as possible while you wait for the ambulance.

For a simple rib injury

Help your child to sit down. Support the arm on the injured side in an arm sling. TAKE YOUR CHILD TO HOSPITAL. Move her as little as possible to prevent internal injury.

≫ *see also*

● Chest wound, *p.56*
● Internal bleeding, *p.55*
● Shock, *p.30*
● Triangular bandages, *p.106*
● Unconscious child, *pp.22–29*

Arm injury

The treatment below is suitable for injuries to the upper arm, forearm, and wrist. Move the injured arm as little as possible.

Place padding around injury

1 Help your child to sit down and, if possible, get him to support his injured arm with his other hand. Place a soft pad between his arm and his chest to protect and cushion the injured limb.

2 Immobilise the injured arm by supporting it in an arm sling. Secure the sling with a reef knot.

Support arm in a sling

Ask him to support injury until sling is secure

» *see also*

● Triangular bandages, p.106

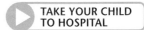 **TAKE YOUR CHILD TO HOSPITAL**

IMPORTANT

● **Do not** attempt to straighten or bend your child's elbow.

Elbow injury

Elbow injuries need early treatment in hospital. Suspect elbow injury if your child is unable to bend his arm; pain is increased by any attempts at movement; there is swelling or bruising around the elbow.

Help your child to lie down and place his arm in the most comfortable position. Support it with cushions if necessary.

Help your child to lie down

Put soft padding between his arm and body

Place injured arm across his body

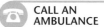 **CALL AN AMBULANCE**

Hand injury

This type of injury can be very painful. There may be several broken bones, and often a joint is dislocated. If your child's hand was crushed there may also be an open wound. Your child will need an X-ray or scan.

 IMPORTANT

● **If there is a wound,** control the bleeding by raising the hand and gently press a clean, non-fluffy dressing or pad over the wound.

Wrap hand in soft padding

Support hand and arm in elevation sling

1 Wrap the injured hand in soft cotton wool padding. Raise your child's hand, supporting it to minimise swelling.

2 Place your child's arm in an elevation sling to reduce swelling and prevent movement of the injured hand.

Trapped fingers

Hold the fingers under cold running water for a few minutes to relieve the pain and minimise swelling. If the fingers still hurt, apply a cold compress (*see p.108*).

Tie broad-fold bandage around arm and body

3 For extra support, tie a broad-fold bandage (*see p.73*) around the arm and body; secure it with a reef knot on the uninjured side.

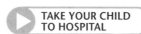 **► TAKE YOUR CHILD TO HOSPITAL**

» *see also*
● Bleeding, *p.44*
● Crush injury, *p.55*
● Triangular bandages, *p.106*

! **IMPORTANT**

● **If** your child has injured her arm, minimise bruising and swelling by supporting the arm in a sling.

Bruises and swellings

After a fall or bump, bruising and swelling may develop rapidly. Resting, cooling, and raising the injury will alleviate symptoms.

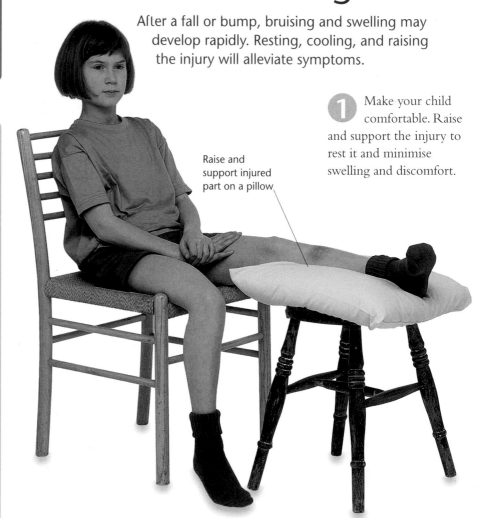

Raise and support injured part on a pillow

1 Make your child comfortable. Raise and support the injury to rest it and minimise swelling and discomfort.

Cold compresses

Applying a cold compress helps minimise swelling and discomfort by reducing blood flow to the area. Make one with a cloth wrung out in cold water, or fill a plastic bag two-thirds full of ice and add a little salt to help the ice melt, then seal. A bag of frozen fruit or vegetables can also be used. (*See p.108.*)

Leave a compress in place for about 30 minutes, ideally uncovered; if you need to secure it, use a loose gauze bandage.

Apply a cold compress to reduce swelling

2 To reduce swelling, hold a cold compress against the injury for 30 minutes (*see left*). If necessary, bandage the compress in place.

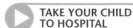
▶ **TAKE YOUR CHILD TO HOSPITAL**

Splinter

There is always a risk of infection with splinters. They are often dirty and the bacteria can be carried deep into the skin. Children are most likely to get splinters in their hands and knees as they crawl on the floor.

IMPORTANT

● **If** your child is not immunised against Tetanus infection, SEEK MEDICAL ADVICE.

● **Do not** poke at the area with a needle to remove the splinter.

● **If** you cannot remove the splinter, or if it breaks off, SEEK MEDICAL ADVICE.

Wash around splinter

1 Clean the area around the splinter thoroughly with soap and warm water.

Sterilise tweezers in a flame

2 Sterilise a pair of tweezers by passing them through a flame. Leave the tweezers to cool. Don't touch the ends or wipe off the soot.

Grasp splinter and pull straight out

Support child's hand

3 Grasp the splinter as close to the skin as possible, and carefully draw it back out at the same angle it went in.

Squeeze area to encourage a little bleeding

4 Squeeze the wound to encourage a little bleeding that will flush out dirt. Wash the area again, pat it dry thoroughly, and cover with a plaster.

≫ see also
● Infected wound, p.48

For an object that cannot be removed

Tell your child to keep his eyes still, and cover his eye with a sterile dressing. Reassure him. TAKE HIM TO HOSPITAL.

» see also
● Eye wound, *p.50*

Object in eye

Tiny hairs or specks of dust on the surface of the eye can be very uncomfortable for a child. However, anything on the surface can generally be washed off easily; try to prevent your child rubbing her eye.

Examine the eye

Separate eyelids gently

Ask her to look right, left, up and down

1 Help your child to sit down, facing the light. Separate the eyelids of the affected eye. Ask her to look right, left, up, and down. Examine her eye thoroughly.

Try to wash out foreign object

Use a bowl to catch water

2 If you can see the foreign object on the surface of the eye, try to wash it off using a jug of clean water. Tilt her head and aim for the inner corner so that water will wash over her eye. Or, try lifting it off with a damp swab or the corner of a handkerchief.

Lift upper eyelid over lower lid

3 If an object is under the eyelid, you can ask an older child to clear it by lifting the upper eyelid over the lower one. You will need to do this for a younger child; if necessary, wrap her in a towel first to stop her grabbing your arms.

Object in ear

Children often push things into their ears. A hard object may become stuck, which can cause pain and temporary deafness; it may even damage the child's ear drum.

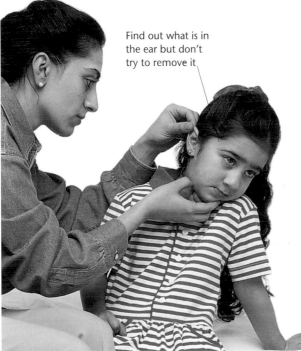

Find out what is in the ear but don't try to remove it

Reassure your child and ask her what she put into her ear. Don't try to remove the object, even if you can see it.

▶ **TAKE YOUR CHILD TO HOSPITAL**

If there is an insect in the ear

If an insect flies or crawls into your child's ear she may be very alarmed.

1 Help her to sit her down. Support her head with the affected ear uppermost.

2 Gently flood the ear with tepid water so that the insect floats out.

IMPORTANT

● **Do** not attempt to remove the object, even if you can see it.

Object in nose

If your child has something stuck in his nose his breathing may be difficult or noisy and his nose may be swollen. Smelly or blood-stained discharge from the nose indicates an object has been present for a while.

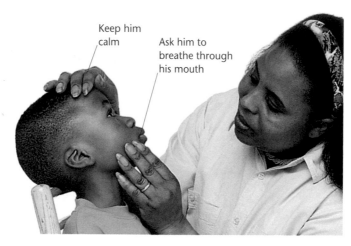

Keep him calm

Ask him to breathe through his mouth

1 Reassure your child and try to find out what he put in his nose. Tell him not to touch it.

2 Tell your child to breathe through his mouth.

▶ **TAKE YOUR CHILD TO HOSPITAL**

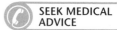 **IMPORTANT**

● **If** the object is sharp or large, don't give your child anything to eat or drink. TAKE YOUR CHILD TO HOSPITAL.

● **If** he has swallowed a battery, TAKE YOUR CHILD TO HOSPITAL.

Swallowed object

Young children often put small objects in their mouths and may swallow them. Most objects will pass straight through the digestive system. Small button batteries are dangerous as they contain corrosive chemicals.

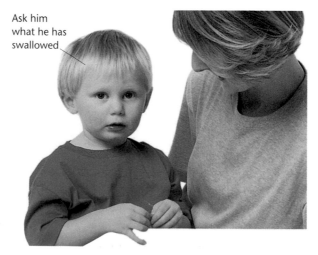

Ask him what he has swallowed

1 Reassure your child. Try to find out what he child has swallowed.

2 If the object is small and smooth like a pebble or a coin, there is little danger.

SEEK MEDICAL ADVICE

Animal bite

The main risk with an animal bite is infection; sharp pointed teeth can carry germs deep into the skin. Severe wounds with torn edges may need stitches. There is a risk of rabies from animals from outside the UK.

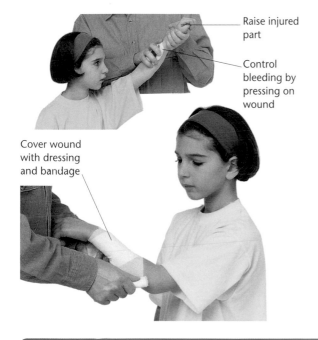

Raise injured part

Control bleeding by pressing on wound

Cover wound with dressing and bandage

1 If bleeding is severe, apply direct pressure over the wound, preferably over a clean dressing or pad. Lift and support the injured part above the level of your child's heart.

2 Cover the wound with a sterile dressing or pad and bandage firmly in place.

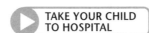
▶ **TAKE YOUR CHILD TO HOSPITAL**

≫ see also
● Bleeding, *p.44*
● Infected wound, *p.48*
● Shock, *p.30*

For a superficial animal bite

1 Wash the wound thoroughly, using soap and warm water. Rinse the wound under running water for at least five minutes to wash away any dirt.

2 Gently, but thoroughly, pat the wound dry with a clean pad or tissue. Cover it with a plaster or a small sterile dressing.

SEEK MEDICAL ADVICE

Wash wound with soap and warm, running water

Dry wound and cover with a plaster

Insect sting

Bee, wasp, or hornet stings can be very alarming for a child, but they are rarely dangerous. Your child will experience a sharp pain followed by soreness, red skin, and slight swelling around the site of the sting.

If sting is in mouth

To reduce swelling, give your child an ice cube to suck or cold water to drink. SEEK MEDICAL ADVICE. If breathing becomes difficult, CALL AN AMBULANCE.

Scrape off a protruding sting

1 If the sting is still in the skin, brush or scrape it off sideways with your fingernail or a plastic card. Do not try to remove it with tweezers as you will inject more poison into your child.

 see also
- Anaphylactic shock, *opposite*

Place a cold compress over area

2 Cool the area with a cold compress to minimise the pain and swelling. Leave the compress in place for about ten minutes, until the pain is relieved. Rest the injured part.

Nettle rash

If your child brushes against nettles he will have a blotchy, red, itchy rash that may frighten him. Reassure him and soothe the rash.

Soothe rash by dabbing with calamine lotion

1 To relieve the itching, dab the rash with cotton wool soaked in calamine lotion.

2 Alternatively, place a cold compress over the rash until the pain is relieved, about ten minutes.

 see also
- Cold compress, *p.108*

Anaphylactic shock

This is a severe allergic reaction that may develop within a few minutes of the injection of a drug, an insect or marine creature sting, or ingestion of a food. It causes constriction of the air passages and swelling of the face and neck that can result in suffocation. Suspect this if your child is anxious with red, blotchy skin, swelling around her face, neck, and eyes, is wheezing, has difficulty breathing, and a rapid pulse.

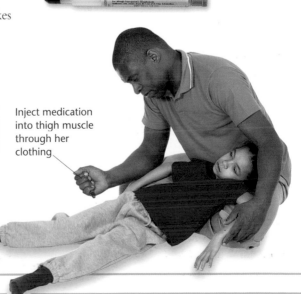

Support her in a position that helps her breathing

CALL AN AMBULANCE

1 Help your child into the position that most relieves her breathing difficulty.

2 Talk to her calmly and reassure her while you wait for the ambulance to arrive.

> **!** **IMPORTANT**
>
> ● **If** your child loses consciousness, open her airway and check breathing. If breathing, place in the recovery position; if not breathing, begin rescue breaths and chest compressions.
>
> ● **If** child has her own medication help her to use it or, if you are trained, give it to her yourself, *see below*.

» *see also*
● Shock, *p.30*

Administering an auto injector

A child with a known allergy may have his own medication to take in case of an attack. This usually takes the form of a syringe or auto-injector of epinephrine (adrenaline) prescribed for the child's own use.

Auto-injector

1 Hold the injector with your fingers and remove the protective grey cap.

Inject medication into thigh muscle through her clothing

2 Holding the injector with your fist, place the black tip firmly against the child's thigh to release the medication. Rub the injection site.

Jellyfish sting

Jellyfish venom is contained in stinging cells that stick to a child's skin. The sting is painful, but not usually serious. A similar reaction is produced by sea anemones and corals.

Cool the affected area with a compress

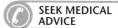
Apply a cold compress against the skin. Leave the compress on the wound for about 10 minutes.

≫ see also

● Anaphylactic shock, p.87

● Cold compresses, p.108

Raise the affected limb

If possible, raise and support the affected part to reduce swelling.

SEEK MEDICAL ADVICE

Weever fish sting

When trodden on, the spines from a weever fish can puncture the skin, causing painful swelling and soreness. The spines can also break off and become embedded in a child's foot.

Immerse her foot in hot water

Immerse the injury in water as hot as your child can bear for at least 30 minutes. Top up as the water cools but be careful not to scald her.

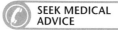
SEEK MEDICAL ADVICE

Snake bite

If your child is bitten by a snake there will be two puncture marks. There may also be redness at the site and he may be feeling sick or vomiting, and be sweating. There may be disturbed vision and difficulty breathing.

Clean and dry the wound

Raise the heart above the level of the bite

☎ **CALL AN AMBULANCE**

1 Help your child to lie down. Keep the heart above the level of the bite area to contain the poison. Gently wash the wound and pat dry with clean swabs.

Apply roller bandage above bite

2 Lightly compress the whole limb above the bite with a roller bandage. If the hand or foot begins to feel numb or cold, loosen the bandage slightly.

Immobilise the limb

3 Immobilise the limb with folded triangular bandages and padding. Reassure your child and keep him still to stop the venom spreading through his body.

⚠ IMPORTANT

● **If** your child develops a severe allergic reaction, treat as for Anaphylactic shock.

● **If** your child loses consciousness, open his airway and check breathing. If breathing, place in the recovery position; if not breathing, begin rescue breaths and chest compressions.

● **Do not** let your child walk about.

● **Do not** apply a tourniquet, cut out the wound, or try to suck out the venom.

● **If** possible give an accurate description of the snake to the medical team to help them with treatment.

⟫ see also

● Anaphylactic shock, *p.87*

● Triangular bandages, *p.106*

● Unconscious baby, *pp.17–21*

● Unconscious child, *p.22–29*

Hypothermia

This develops if the body temperature falls. Deep hypothermia, where the body temperature falls very low, is extremely serious. An older child is most likely to develop it outside in poor weather conditions, or after falling into cold water. For babies, see opposite. Your child is suffering from hypothermia if she is shivering and has cold, pale, dry skin; she is listless or confused and is losing consciousness; and she has slow, shallow breathing and a weakening pulse.

Wrap her in warm towels

Give her a warm bath

1 Give your child a warm bath, if she is able to climb in herself. When her skin colour has returned to normal, help her out, dry her quickly, and wrap her in warm towels or blankets.

Cover her head with a hat

Warm her hands with gloves

2 Dress your child with warm clothes and put her to bed, covered with plenty of blankets. Cover her head with a hat and make sure that the room is warm. Stay with her.

SEEK MEDICAL ADVICE

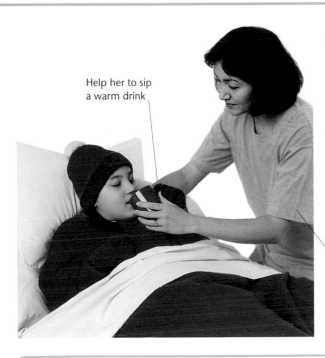

Help her to sip a warm drink

3 Give your child a warm drink and some high-energy foods, such as chocolate. Do not leave her alone until you are sure that her colour and temperature have returned to normal.

Stay with her until colour and temperature have returned to normal

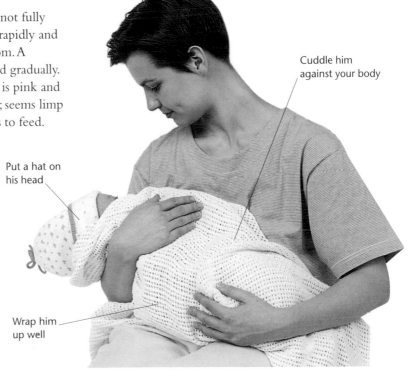

» *see also*
● Unconscious baby, *pp.17–21*
● Unconscious child, *p.22–29*

Hypothermia in babies

A baby's temperature regulation is not fully developed. He can lose body heat rapidly and develop hypothermia in a cold room. A hypothermic baby must be warmed gradually. Suspect hypothermia if your baby: is pink and healthy looking but skin feels cold; seems limp and unusually quiet; and he refuses to feed.

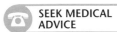 **SEEK MEDICAL ADVICE**

1 Warm a baby gradually. Take him into a warm room. Wrap him in blankets.

2 Put a hat on his head and cuddle him against your body so that he is warmed by your body heat.

Cuddle him against your body

Put a hat on his head

Wrap him up well

If recovery is slow or skin broken

If there are any open wounds, the frozen skin is broken, or the colour does not return rapidly, cover the area with a soft gauze dressing and bandage it lightly in place. TAKE YOUR CHILD TO HOSPITAL.

Frostbite

If children are exposed to extreme weather conditions, the tissues of the fingers and toes may freeze. Your child may have frostbite if she has pins and needles in her fingers or toes with numbness and hard, stiff skin that is turning white and waxy. Shelter your child before treating her.

Remove clothing from affected area carefully

1 Take your child into a warm shelter before you start treatment. Help her to sit down, then very gently remove her shoes and socks.

Take her gloves off very carefully

Warm hands with her own body heat, under armpits

2 Remove gloves and any rings. Undo her coat. Tell her to put her hands under her armpits to warm them with her own body heat.

Use your body heat to thaw feet

3 When your child's feet or toes are frozen, raise her feet to reduce swelling. Place her feet in your own armpits to warm her toes.

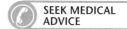

SEEK MEDICAL ADVICE

Heat exhaustion

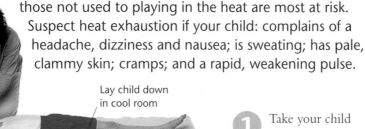

This may develop in hot, humid weather and is caused by dehydration. Children who are unwell, particularly with diarrhoea and vomiting, and those not used to playing in the heat are most at risk. Suspect heat exhaustion if your child: complains of a headache, dizziness and nausea; is sweating; has pale, clammy skin; cramps; and a rapid, weakening pulse.

 IMPORTANT

- **Seek** medical advice even if your child recovers quickly.

- **If** your child does not recover quickly he could delevop heatstroke.

- **If** your child loses consciousness, open his airway and check breathing. If breathing, place in the recovery position; if not breathing, begin rescue breaths and chest compressions. CALL AN AMBULANCE.

Lay child down in cool room

Put folded towel or cushion under his head

1 Take your child into the shade or into a cool room. Help him to lie down.

Raise his legs

2 Raise and support your child's legs on some pillows. This improves blood supply to the brain. Encourage him to rest quietly.

Give him as much cool water as he can manage

3 Help your child to sit up and sip as much cool water as he can manage. Later give him cool salty water solution (made up of 5ml/1 teaspoon of salt per litre of fluid) or diluted fruit juice, to replace salt lost from the body.

 SEEK MEDICAL ADVICE

» *see also*
- Heatstroke, *p.94*
- Unconscious baby, *pp.17–21*
- Unconscious child, *p.22–29*

ⓘ IMPORTANT

● If a baby or very young child develops heatstroke, undress him completely in a cool room.

● If your child loses consciousness, open his airway and check breathing. If breathing, place in the recovery position; if not breathing, begin rescue breaths and chest compressions.

Heatstroke

This is a serious condition that develops if the body becomes overheated in hot surroundings. Treat for heatstroke if your child: develops a sudden headache; is confused; has hot, flushed, dry skin; has a full bounding pulse; is losing consciousness; has a temperature of over 40°C (104°F).

Help your child to lie down in a cool room

Remove his clothes

1 Help your child to lie down in a cool place and remove all outer clothing. Put a folded towel or pillow under his head and reassure him.

☎ CALL AN AMBULANCE

Sponge his face and body with tepid water

2 Sponge down your child repeatedly with cold or tepid water. Leave his skin damp and let it dry in the air.

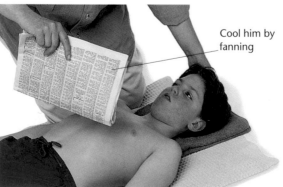

Cool him by fanning

3 Fan your child by hand or with an electric fan to help bring his temperature down. Continue cooling until his temperature down to 38°C (100.4°F).

≫ see also

● Unconscious baby, pp.17–21

● Unconscious child, p.22–29

Sunburn

Sunburn is red, itchy, and tender. Babies and young children are very vulnerable: keep them in shade; apply sun block; put on a hat and cover with protective clothing in hot weather.

Give him cold water to sip

Take him into shade

Apply cooling cream to reduce discomfort

1 Move your child into the shade or into a cool room and give him a cold drink.

2 Apply calamine cream or a special after-sun cream to soothe the skin. Make sure it is a cream that you *know* your child is not allergic to.

IMPORTANT

● **If** there is blistering, SEEK MEDICAL ADVICE.

● **If** your child is restless, flushed, dizzy, or has a temperature or headache, he may have heatstroke.

see also

● Heat exhaustion, *p.93*

● Heatstroke, *opposite*

Heat rash

This a prickly, red rash that develops particularly around the sweat glands on the chest and back and under the arms.

1 Help your child to sit down in a cool room and undress her. Sponge the affected area with cool water.

2 Pat her almost dry with a soft towel, leaving the skin slightly damp. Apply calamine cream to the rash.

Sponge her down

Leave her skin to dry off in the air

IMPORTANT

● **If** your baby develops heat rash, remove some of her clothes to cool her, or bathe her in tepid water. Dry her gently, leaving her skin slightly damp.

● **If** the rash has not faded after 12 hours, or if she develops a raised temperature, SEEK MEDICAL ADVICE.

! IMPORTANT

● **If** your baby is under three months old, you should not give her paracetamol syrup, unless you are advised to do so by your doctor.

● **If** your child is very hot, take as many clothes off as possible.

● **If** your child complains of a severe headache, suspect meningitis. SEEK MEDICAL ADVICE.

● **Fever** can also be caused by too much sun, see heatstroke.

Fever

A body temperature that is above 37°C (98.6°F) indicates fever. An infection is the usual cause. A moderate fever is not harmful, but a temperature above 40°C (104°F) can be dangerous, particularly in babies and very young children. Your child has a fever if she: has a raised temperature; looks very pale; complains she feels cold with goose pimples; is shivering, with chattering teeth. As the fever advances she will have hot, flushed skin, be sweating, and have a headache.

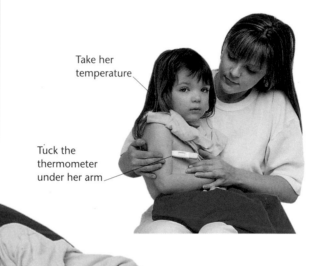

Take her temperature

Tuck the thermometer under her arm

1 Take your child's temperature. Lift your child's arm and tuck the pointed end of the thermometer into her armpit. Fold her arm over her chest and leave the thermometer in place for the recommended time.

Leave a drink beside her

2 Make your child comfortable on a bed or sofa, but do not cover her. To help bring down her temperature, make sure she has plenty of water or diluted fruit juice to drink.

3 You can give her the recommended dose of paracetamol syrup to help reduce her temperature.

>> see also

● Febrile seizures, *p.32*
● Heatstroke, *p.94*
● Meningitis, *opposite*

Give her recommended dose of paracetamol syrup

Meningitis

This is a life-threatening infection affecting the tissues that surround the brain. In the early stages your child will have a flu-like illness with a high temperature. He may tell you he has cold hands and feet and limb pain, and he may have mottled or very pale skin. As the infection develops he is likely to have a headache, neck stiffness, and begin vomiting. His eyes may be sensitive to light and he will become increasingly drowsy. Later, a red or purple rash may develop that does not disappear if you press it.

! IMPORTANT

● **If** there is any delay contacting medical advice, TAKE YOUR CHILD TO HOSPITAL or CALL AN AMBULANCE.

● **Do not** let him get too hot.

Child may complain that light hurts his eyes

1 If your child has a high fever and a flu-like illness, monitor him carefully. If light hurts his eyes, let him rest in a darker room and monitor for other signs. Treat fever. Give him plenty of fluids to drink and the recommended dose of paracetamol syrup.

SEEK MEDICAL ADVICE

Meningitis rash will remain visible if you press a glass against it

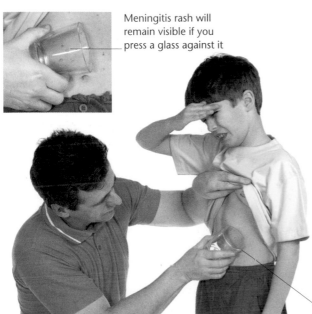

2 Check your child's body for signs of a rash. If you see any spots, press a glass gently against them. If you can still see the spots through the glass,

 CALL AN AMBULANCE

》》 *see also*
● Febrile seizures, *p.32*
● Fever, *opposite*

Press side of a glass against the rash

Vomiting and diarrhoea

A baby or child who is suffering repeated vomiting and/or diarrhoea can become dehydrated very quickly. It is important to replace lost fluids by giving your child sips of cooled, boiled water. Don't give a baby or child milk unless you are breastfeeding.

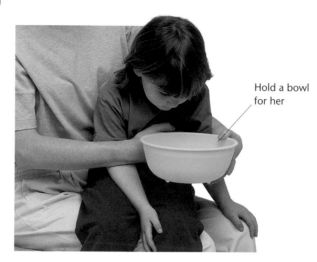

Hold a bowl for her

1 If your child is being sick, hold her over a bowl. Support her upper body with your free hand while she is being sick. Reassure her. Once she has stopped vomiting, wipe her face and around her mouth with a sponge or cloth wrung out in tepid water.

Give her water to drink

2 Give her drinks of water to replace any fluid loss and to remove the unpleasant taste. Encourage her to sip each drink slowly.

3 Let her rest quietly, in bed if she wants to. Make sure the bowl is still at hand in case she is sick again, and give a fresh drink of water.

Stomachache

This is generally caused by a stomach upset or similar minor condition. Occasionally it results from inflammation of the abdominal organs.

Prop her up against cushions or pillows

Provide a bowl if she feels sick

Give her a covered hot-water to hold

1 Make your child comfortable on a sofa or bed. If she is having difficulty breathing, help her to lie back against cushions or pillows. She may want to be sick so leave a container near her.

2 Warmth may help to relieve the pain. Fill a hot-water bottle – it must be covered – and give it to your child to hold against her stomach. Avoid giving her anything to eat until pain subsides.

Appendicitis

Inflammation of the appendix is rare under the age of two but it may affect older, especially teenage, children. Suspect appendicitis if your child complains of waves of pain in the middle of his abdomen or of acute pain settling in the right lower abdomen. He may also have a raised temperature, no appetite, nausea, vomiting, and diarrhoea.

Suspected appendicitis must be treated promptly. Help your child to lie down. Do not give him anything to eat or drink.

Pain starts here

Pain settles here

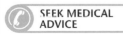
SEEK MEDICAL ADVICE

Pressure-change earache

This may happen on plane journeys, particularly when taking off or landing, or when travelling through tunnels. To make the ears "pop" so that the pressure is relieved, an older child should close her mouth, hold her nose and blow down it. Sucking a sweet may also help.

Earache

This is most commonly caused by an ear infection following a cold or 'flu. Earache can be the result of a child putting something in her ear.

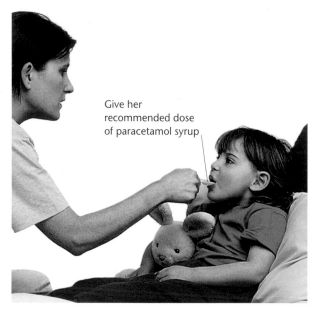

Give her recommended dose of paracetamol syrup

1 Make your child comfortable. Help her to sit up supported by pillows or cushions if lying down makes the earache worse. You can give the recommended dose of paracetamol syrup.

2 Applying heat may help to soothe the pain. Prepare a covered hot–water bottle and tell your child to lie down with her painful ear against it.

Provide a covered hot-water bottle to place against her ear

Prop her up with pillows

Toothache

A toddler who complains of toothache may have a new tooth coming through. An older child may have tooth decay or an infection.

Give her recommended dose of paracetamol syrup

Give her a covered hot-water bottle to lie against

1 Arrange an early appointment with your child's dentist. Meanwhile, give her the recommended dose of paracetamol syrup to relieve the pain.

2 Lying flat, or propped on pillows or cushions, with a covered hot-water bottle against the affected cheek may help relieve the pain.

Cramp

Cramp is a painful muscle spasm that often affects the foot and calf muscles. You can relieve the pain by massaging and stretching the affected muscles.

1 Help your child to sit down then raise her leg and straighten her knee. Ease her toes upwards to flex the foot.

2 Gently but firmly knead the affected muscles with your fingertips until the spasm has passed completely.

Ease her foot upwards and forwards

Straighten her leg

Support her foot in your hand

A well stocked first aid kit

- Disposable gloves
- 1 small roller bandage
- 1 large roller bandage
- 1 small conforming bandage
- 1 large conforming bandage
- Scissors and tweezers
- Calamine cream
- Pack of gauze swabs
- 2 triangular bandages
- Hypoallergenic tape
- 2 sterile pads
- Waterproof plasters
- 1 finger bandage and applicator
- 1 sterile dressing with bandage

First aid kit

Keep first aid kits in your car and in your home. You can buy kits ready made up. You may want to add extra dressings and bandages or specialist plasters – blister plasters, for example. Make sure the first aid box is readily accessible and easy to identify, and check the contents regularly. Don't keep medicines in the first aid box; they should be locked in a medicine cabinet. A well stocked kit might contain the articles shown below. See p.108 for other useful equipment.

Scissors

Tweezers

Calamine cream or lotion

Sterile non-adhesive pad

Dressings

Plasters (adhesive dressings) are used for minor wounds. Keep several different sizes and shapes., including a selection of larger sterile dressings for more serious wounds.

Plasters

Gauze swabs

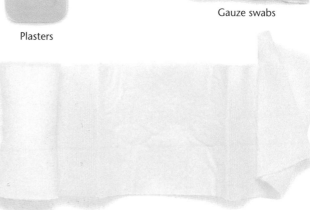

Sterile dressing with bandage

Bandages

Keep a variety of bandages to secure dressings and support injured joints. Conforming bandages shape themselves to the contours of the body and so are easy to use. Triangular bandages can be used as slings and for broad- and narrow-fold bandages.

Hypoallergenic tape for securing dressings

Small conforming bandage

Large conforming bandage

Applicator

Clip secures bandage

Crepe roller bandage

Finger bandage

Large roller bandage

Safety pins

Folded triangular bandage

Other useful items

A variety of household items are invaluable for first aid emergencies. If you don't have exactly the right materials, you can improvise successfully. Keep the following articles to hand.

FLANNEL

Use a flannel soaked in water to make a cold compress as well as clean up a child after an incident.

SHEETS AND PILLOW CASES

A clean cotton sheet or pillowcase makes an excellent loose protective covering for burns.

KITCHEN FILM

Plastic kitchen film can be used to dress burns and seal chest wounds.

PLASTIC BAGS

A clean plastic bag can be put over a burned foot or hand and lightly secured with bandages or tape. Always cool the burn first.

Dressings

Covering a wound helps the blood-clotting process and prevents infection. Dressings should not be fluffy and must be large enough to cover the wound and area around it. Wash your hands before applying dressings and wear disposable gloves if possible. If blood soaks through a dressing, place another on top. Make sure bandages are not too tight (see opposite).

Plaster

Remove wrapping and, holding the pad over the wound, peel back the protective strips. Press the ends and edges down.

Sterile pad

Place pad on wound

Cover with a bandage

Secure bandage with tape

1 Place the dressing pad shiny-side down directly over the child's wound.

2 Secure the pad with a bandage, working from below the injury up the limb.

3 Secure the end of the bandage with strips of hypoallergenic tape.

Sterile dressing with bandage

Place pad over wound

Wind long bandage around limb

Tie reef knot over pad

1 Hold the bandage either side of the dressing pad, and place the pad over the wound.

2 Leaving the short end hanging, wind the other end around the limb to cover dressing.

3 Tie the two ends of the bandage in a reef knot (see p.106) directly over the pad.

Bandaging

Use bandages to secure dressings, to help control bleeding, and to support injuries. Roller bandages can be used for any part of the body; conforming bandages are especially useful for bandaging joints or head wounds as they mould themselves to the shape of the body.

Check circulation

Do not apply a bandage too tightly – it will impair the circulation. To check, press on your child's nail or a patch of skin, then release pressure. The colour should return rapidly. If it does not, loosen the bandages.

Roller bandage

Start at wrist

Wind bandage up the limb

Secure end with tape

1 Place the end of the bandage on the arm below the injury and hold the bandage roll in your other hand.

2 Still supporting the injured limb, wind the bandage around the arm, working up the limb. Stop above the injury.

3 Make two straight turns to finish. Secure the end with tape. Check circulation in your child's fingers (*see above*).

Hand bandage

Start at wrist

Bandage in figure of eight

Secure at wrist with tape

1 Supporting the injured hand, hold the end of the bandage on the wrist and make two straight turns around the wrist.

2 Take the bandage across the back of the hand to the base of the little finger. Then take it around the palm, up between the

thumb and forefinger, and across the back of the hand to the wrist. Repeat the figure of eight to cover the hand. Check circulation.

Triangular bandages

These are sold singly in sterile packs or can be made from a square of strong fabric folded diagonally in half. Triangular bandages are used for broad-fold and narrow-fold bandages (*see p.73*) or slings. Arm slings support injured arms or wrists, or take weight off an injured shoulder. Elevation slings are used for arm and upper body injuries where bleeding, pain, or swelling need to be reduced. Use a reef knot to secure slings as it lies flat so is more comfortable.

Arm sling

Drape long edge of triangle on uninjured side

1 Place the bandage between your child's arm and chest, easing one end up around the back of his neck on the injured side.

Tie a reef knot at shoulder

Bring lower end up over forearm

2 Take the lower end of the bandage up over your child's forearm to the end at the shoulder and tie a reef knot (see below) just below the shoulder.

Make the reef knot comfortable

Tuck in surplus fabric at elbow

3 Fold in the surplus fabric at the corner near the elbow and pin it to the bandage.

Tying a reef knot

1 Cross the left end (yellow) over the right (blue) one.

2 Then take the yellow end under the blue.

3 Pass the yellow over the blue and through gap.

4 Pull the ends firmly to secure the knot.

Elevation sling

Rest fingertips on shoulder of uninjured side

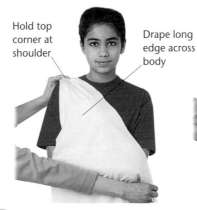

Hold top corner at shoulder

Drape long edge across body

Scoop bandage up around elbow

1 Bring the arm on the injured side across your child's chest. Ask her to support her elbow.

2 Lay bandage over child's arm, with longest edge on the uninjured side. Hold the top corner.

3 Support the child's arm and fold long edge of bandage in under injured arm.

Tie ends just in front of shoulder on uninjured side

4 Bring the lower end up around her back, holding the elbow securely in the fabric. Tie a reef knot (opposite) just below the shoulder and tuck the ends in.

Gather slack fabric at elbow and tuck in behind

OR

Pin slack fabric to front of sling

5 Secure the sling by twisting the excess fabric and tucking it in at the elbow or fold and pin in place.

Finished sling raises, immobilises, and supports the injury

Other useful first aid equipment

You should keep your first aid kit well stocked (*see p.102*) at home and in the car. However, there are other items that can be useful in an emergency, from specialist equipment such as plastic face masks for resuscitation and survival blankets, to everyday items around the home.

Additional equipment

- Plastic face shields or face masks, will protect you and a casualty when you are giving rescue breaths.
- If you have a note pad and pen or pencil you can write down important information about a child's condition to give to the emergency services.
- Keep a plastic or foil emergency survival blanket or bag in your car at all times.
- Always carry a warning triangle in your car and place it in the road behind the car in the event of a breakdown or crash.
- Keep a torch beside your home first aid kit (for use in the event of a power failure), and in your car; check and replace the batteries regularly.

Useful liquids

- Use vinegar to treat a tropical jellyfish sting (*see p.88*). Pour the vinegar over the sting and surrounding area; it neutralises the effect of the sting and prevents it from spreading.
- Beer or milk can be used to cool a burn if there is no cold water available (*see p.58*).
- Milk stops a knocked-out adult tooth drying out while you get the child to a dentist (*see p.53*).

Making a cold compress

- Packs of frozen vegetables such as peas or fruit such as raspberries or currants make ideal ice packs. They can be moulded to the shape of the body and stay cool for a long time.
- Make your own ice pack using a sandwich or freezer bag. Fill the plastic bag two-thirds full of ice cubes, add a little salt to make ice melt faster, then seal the bag. Wrap it in a cloth before putting on your child.
- Soak a flannel in water, wring out the excess, and place it over an injury.

Frozen peas in a plastic bag

Improvised slings

If your child injures her shoulder, arm, or hand, you can make an improvised sling to support the injury until she receives medical treatment.

- Undo a coat or shirt button and tuck the hand of the injured arm inside the fastening.

- Pin your child's sleeve up on the opposite side of his chest.

Support injury in coat fastening

Pin sleeve to coat

Safety at home

Most accidents occur at home and over half involve children under the age of five. Many accidents are preventable if you:

- Plan the layout and position of objects and furniture at home with child safety in mind.
- Make sure that all windows are closed or inaccessible (don't leave chairs beside them).
- Never confuse containers by putting a dangerous substance, such as bleach, in a bottle that used to contain a harmless drink.
- Install smoke alarms, fire guards, and safety gates in your home.
- Never pretend that medicines and pills are special sweets to encourage a child to take medication. Keep medicines locked away.
- Check for hazards when visiting friends and ask if you can move sharp or breakable objects.
- Teach your child basic safety rules.

Fire

If fire breaks out at home, it could be a matter of minutes before smoke overcomes you.

- Fit smoke detectors throughout your home. If your home is on one level, fit a detector between the sitting room and the bedrooms. If your house is on two or more levels, fit one detector at the foot of the stairs and another outside the bedrooms upstairs. If you live in an apartment block there should be detectors in all communal areas.
- Check and replace smoke detector batteries regularly.
- Have an escape plan (*see p. 11*). Make sure the whole family knows what to do if there is a fire; practise the fire drill with your children: shout "fire"; set off the smoke detector; tell everyone to drop to the floor and crawl to the nearest exit from the rooms; shut each door behind you; arrange a point in the garden for example, where the children should wait together.
- Don't go back for pets or treasured possessions.

Electricity

Protect your child from electric shock (*see p. 12*).

- Cover sockets: put heavy furniture in front of them, or fit plastic covers.
- Put only one or two plugs into each socket – overloading can cause sockets to overheat.
- Wire plugs correctly – follow instructions and check that you have the right fuse.
- Replace worn or damaged flexes – a child may try to chew protuding wires.
- Tidy up trailing wires to prevent tripping hazards.
- Unplug electrical appliances at night, particularly the televisions and computers.
- Fit an RCD (residual current device) to power tools.

Gas

Find out where your gas tap is in case there is a leak. If you smell gas:

- Don't turn lights or electric switches on or off – there may be a spark, which could cause an explosion.
- Don't light matches or cigarettes.
- Turn off the gas.
- Open the windows.
- Call the gas company.

Teach your child to recognise hazards

Hall and stairs

The staircase is not a safe place for your child to play (*see below*).

- Make sure that toys are not left on the stairs for you to trip over.
- Put a light in your hall or on the landing so that your child can see if he gets up at night.

If you don't want the area too light, use a low-watt bulb. Never cover a lamp with a cloth as the cloth can easily catch fire.

- Don't let your child play on the landings or stairs of a communal area in flats as the banisters may have large gaps between them.

Front and back doors

- Never leave your front door open.
- Don't let your child answer the door to callers.
- Put the door catch out of reach of small children. If your toddler can reach the catch, fix an additional bolt higher up the door and keep the door bolted.
- Stick plastic safety film over glass doors if the glass is within 80cm (2ft 8in) of the floor; this prevents the glass splintering if it is broken. Better still, fit toughened or laminated glass.
- Put stickers over the glass to make it more noticeable, especially for young children.

Floors

Tiled, polished, or hessian-covered floors can be very slippery for toddlers and running children.

- Put non-slip webbing under rugs.
- Keep hall floors free of toys and clutter.
- Check fitted carpets regularly for holes or loose carpet that might trip you or your toddler.

Stairs

A child is not co-ordinated enough to be able to walk downstairs safely until he is at least three years old.

- Fit stair gates at the foot of the stairs and across the upper landing or across your child's bedroom doorway (stair gates at the top of the stairs can be a trip hazard). Stair gates should comply with British Standard EN 1930:2000 so the bars are no more than 6.5cm (2½in) apart. Always open the gate; never climb over it as your child will copy you.
- Check your banisters regularly: the handrail and posts should be secured. Posts should not be too far apart – anything wider than 6.5cm (2½in) apart should be boarded up. Don't let your child climb banisters.
- Replace loose or worn carpet or steps. They are trip hazards.

Keep the stairgate closed

Sitting room

While your children are very young, try to arrange the room so that both children and your valuables are kept out of harm's way.
● If you have a balcony, block up gaps in the railings with hardboard and ensure that the balcony is too high for your child to climb.
● Fit toughened glass in patio doors if the glass is within 80cm (2ft 8in) of the floor.

Carpets and curtains
● Check that there are no areas of carpet or rug that have holes or turned-up edges; either you or your child could trip up.
● Wind up and tuck away all curtain ties and pull cords for blinds. Children can be strangled if they get caught in dangling cords.

Fireplaces and heaters
● Don't leave matches or cigarette lighters where your child can reach them.
● Cover all fires with a fireguard. Fix the guard to the wall to prevent your child pulling it over.
● Use a spark-guard as well as a fireguard for open solid fuel fires as an additional precaution.
● Never use the fireguard as a shelf or clothes airer.

Electrical equipment
● Fix wiring to the skirting board.
● Run long flexes behind furniture so that your child can't trip or pull on them.
● Cover unused plug sockets with safety covers.
● Check that old flexes are not worn.
● Ensure that the TV stand is secure and cannot be pulled over.

Surfaces and furniture
● Place house plants out of reach of young children. Some house plants are poisonous, and others can scratch or produce allergic reactions if touched.
● Do not place breakable or heavy objects on low tables. Set them well back from the edges of surfaces such as window sills or mantelpieces.
● Remove glass-topped tables and put corner protectors on sharp table corners.
● Don't leave hot drinks, alcohol, glasses, cigarettes, matches, or lighters on low surfaces, such as coffee tables, where your child can reach them.
● Keep alcohol in a locked cupboard.
● Never leave a cigarette burning in an ashtray on the arm of a sofa or armchair.
● Replace old foam furniture; it can be lethal in a fire as it releases toxic fumes as soon as it is alight.

Ensure bookcases are secured to the wall

Sofas and armchairs must have fire-resistant fillings and coverings

Kitchen

This is the busiest part of your house, where you spend a lot of time with your children.

- Never hold baby or child in your arms when you are cooking or carrying a hot drink.

Doors

- Cover any glass panels within 80cm (2ft 8in) of the floor with safety film, to stop glass shattering or splintering if broken.Or fit toughened glass.
- Put some colourful stickers on the glass door panels to alert your child.

Floors

- Don't let your child play on the area of floor between you and the work surface or where you could trip over him.
- Avoid bumps and falls by wiping up spills immediately.
- Remove pet food bowls after use and keep that part of the floor scrupulously clean.
- Keep a box for tidying away toys and clutter.

Wastebins

- Discourage toddlers from rummaging in the wastebin.
- Put sharp-edged cans and lids or broken glass straight into the dustbin outside.
- Keep the wastebin in a cupboard with a child-resistant safety catch.

> **! IMPORTANT**
>
> - Keep a fire blanket in the kitchen for smothering flare-ups. If you want to buy a fire extinguisher, consult your local fire brigade to find out which is the most appropriate type. Check them regularly. For more on fires, *see p.11* and *p.109.*

Babies in the kitchen

Stay with your child when he is eating in case he chokes

BOTTLES AND FOOD

- Sterilise all your baby's feeding equipment, or put it in a dishwasher.
- Don't leave a prepared feed standing at room temperature, and don't keep the remains of the last feed. Warmed and reheated feeds are breeding grounds for bacteria.
- Don't heat bottles in a microwave.

HIGHCHAIRS

- Always use the safety harness.
- Never leave the chair where your baby can reach out and pull objects down from a surface.
- Never leave your child unattended in a highchair.

PLAY

- Put your baby in a playpen away from the cooking area, or put a gate across the doorway so he can see you but is out of harm's way.
- Keep him out of range of any spills from the cooker.

Attach a safety harness to the clips on either side of the chair

Choose a stable highchair with widely spaced legs

Tables and work surfaces

- Always be aware of your child's reach and keep all heavy, breakable, or sharp objects well back from the edges of work surfaces.
- Keep stools or chairs away from tables and kitchen work surfaces to prevent a young child from climbing up on them.
- Tuck flexes of kettles, toasters, blenders, and irons out of reach. Choose a curly flex for your kettle if possible. It is not only boiling, steaming kettles that pose a hazard: the water in a kettle is still hot enough to scald 15 minutes after boiling.
- Leave electrical appliances unplugged when they are not in use.
- Avoid using a tablecloth. It is tempting for a crawling baby or toddler to use it to pull himself up, bringing anything on the table down upon his head. Use table mats instead, or secure the cloth with clips.
- Do not put your baby on a table or work surface when he is in a car seat or bouncing cradle: he could easily fall off.

Cupboards and drawers

- Put safety catches on cupboards and drawers, particularly those containing: matches, lighters, knives, scissors, and cutlery; heavy pots, pans, or china; dried food, such as lentils or pasta, which may be a choking hazard; bottles containing alcohol; medicines; cleaning materials, such as washing powder, or dishwasher detergent, even if fitted with "child-resistant" lids.

Fridges

Food poisoning can be caused by poor food storage. Take precautions to minimise risks:

- Keep cooked meat and poultry on a separate shelf from uncooked meat. Cover uncooked meat with kitchen film.
- Don't store food in open tins; tip leftovers into a clean container, cover, and put in the fridge.
- Check food regularly to see that nothing is kept beyond the "use-by" date.

Cookers

Your child is obviously at risk of burns and scalds from hot fat or boiling water when you are preparing food.

- You can buy safety guards, but remember that a child can still poke fingers through some types and be burnt by hot hobs or gas rings.
- Always keep your child away from oven doors; they can get very hot while the oven is in use and will stay hot for some time afterwards. A crawling baby or toddler is particularly at risk. Try to teach your child what "hot" means so that he understands a warning.
- Keep matches and lighters well out of reach in a cupboard fitted with a safety catch.

Use the back rings if possible

If using front rings, point pan handles towards back of cooker

Fit child-resistant safety catches on all cupboard doors and drawers

Washing and drying machines

- Keep small hands away from the glass door; it may get hot while the machine is on.
- Ensure the door is closed when the machines are not in use. Your toddler may try to climb inside or even fill it with toys.

Bedrooms

The cupboards and drawers in bedrooms are always exciting places for toddlers and young children. Make sure any potentially hazardous items are out of reach, as you may not always know when your child will decide to go exploring on his own.

Baby's cots

- Make sure the cot is deep enough to prevent your baby from climbing out – at least 50cm (1ft 8in) from the top of the mattress to the top of the cot.

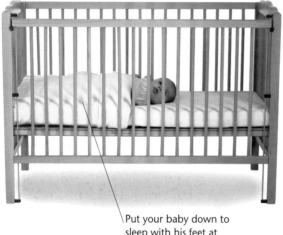

Put your baby down to sleep with his feet at the base of the cot

- Bar spaces must be between 2.5 and 6cm (1–2½in) wide to prevent your baby's head from being trapped.
- The mattress must fit the cot with a gap of less than 3cm (1½in) around the side or the baby's head could become trapped between the cot side and the mattress.
- Don't use a cot that has been handed down through generations; it is unlikely to meet safety standards.
- Don't use a pillow for a baby under one year: it could suffocate him. If you need to raise his head, put a pillow underneath the mattress.
- Use a sheet and cellular blankets rather than a duvet until your baby is one year old. Your baby could overheat or suffocate under a duvet.
- Always put your baby to sleep on his back with his feet at the foot of the cot to lessen the risk of cot death.
- Remove toys from the cot as soon as your baby can sit up because he could use them to climb out.
- Once your child starts trying to climb out of the cot, transfer him to a bed.

Changing areas

- Keep all changing equipment in one area so that you never have to leave your baby alone on the changing mat. He will be safest on the floor, but if you have a changing table, remember that he might roll off if left even for a moment.
- Do not have shelves above the changing area in case something falls off onto your child.
- Keep dangling mobiles out of his reach.
- If you use talcum powder, sprinkle it on your hands and rub them together before applying it to avoid creating a cloud of dust around your baby.

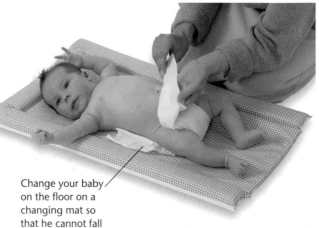

Change your baby on the floor on a changing mat so that he cannot fall

Children's bedrooms

- Don't use a bed guard when your toddler first moves to a bed; if you think he may fall out, put cushions on the floor beside the bed.
- A top bunk bed is not recommended for children under the age of six.
- Top bunk beds must have safety rails on both sides and any gaps in the railings or between the top of the mattress and the bottom of the safety rail should be no more than 6–7.5cm (2½–3in).
- Never let young children play on the top bunk.
- Remove toys from the floor by the bed at night.
- Ensure no wires the child can pull are near bed.

Avoid feather pillows and duvets as they can provoke allergies

WINDOWS

Make sure your child can't climb out of the window. He is in danger even if his room is on the ground floor.
- Fix a safety catch, but make sure the window can be opened easily in the event of a fire.
- Try not to place a piece of furniture below a window because it may encourage your child to climb up.

TOYS *(see also p.117)*
- Keep toys that are unsuitable for very young children separate from others. This way you can easily put them out of reach if your child is sharing a room with a younger child, or if you have young visitors.

Put non-slip webbing under rugs

Your bedroom

- Medicines and pills should never be left beside your bed, or on a dressing table. Put them out of sight and out of reach, preferably in a locked cupboard.
- Scissors and sewing equipment should be kept in a drawer or cupboard with a safety catch.
- Perfume, hairspray, and makeup can be harmful if sprayed or rubbed in the eyes, or swallowed, so keep them out of reach or in a drawer with a safety catch. Make-up spills can also stain a carpet.
- Never leave a china cup or a glass on the floor by your bed, especially at night. If your child is in your bed he could roll out onto the cup or the glass.

Bathroom

Your child may be at risk from falls, drowning, or poisoning in the bathroom. Keep the door shut at all times to discourage him from going in. If you install a bolt to the bathroom door, fix it towards the top of the door to prevent a young child locking himself in.

Showers
- Keep a constant check on the temperature of the water.
- Use non-slip mats in the shower and on the bathroom floor.
- Fix safety film on a glass shower door so that glass is held in place in case of an accident.

Baths
- Check the temperature of the water before your child gets into the bath. Put your elbow in the water; if it is too hot for your elbow it is too hot for your child. A child can be badly scalded by hot bathwater.
- Fit thermostatic mixing valves to the hot taps to limit the temperature of water from the tap.
- Place non-slip mats in the bath and on the floor beside the bath.

- Don't let babies or toddlers play with the bath taps.
- Never leave a young child or baby alone in the bath (or in the care of another child). A baby can drown in just 2.5cm (1in) of water. If you need to answer the door or telephone, take your baby with you.

Cupboards and cabinets
- Store bathroom chemicals and other potential poisons, such as toilet cleaners and bleach, out of reach in a cupboard with a safety catch.
- Keep other hazards, such as make-up, aftershave, razors, nail scissors, and any medicines or glass containers, out of reach in a locked medicine cabinet.

Toilets
- Use a special child toilet seat adaptor and step for toddlers so that they can keep their balance more easily and so feel more secure.
- Keep the toilet seat closed.
- Don't use block toilet cleaners that a young child could pull out and chew.
- Never use toilet cleaners as well as bleach as this will produce toxic fumes.
- If your toddler uses a potty, keep it clean, but never leave bleach or cleaning agents inside it.

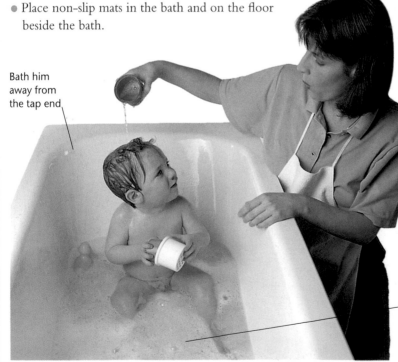

Bath him away from the tap end

Use a non-slip mat in the bath

Toys and playthings

If you have children of different ages in your home, keep their toys in separate boxes. In particular, keep toys with small parts away from younger children. All toys should bear the CE safety mark.

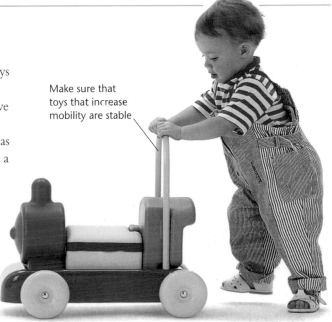

Give your child non-toxic paints to play with

Choosing toys

- Buy toys that are appropriate for the age of your child, and buy from a reputable source.
- Don't give your child anything to play with that has sharp edges, or is made of thin, rigid plastic.
- Give him non-toxic paints or crayons.
- Don't buy your child old second-hand toys: they may be broken or covered in paint containing lead.
- Avoid novelty toys that are not designed to be played with by young children: look out for warnings on the packaging.

Check sets of building blocks for small pieces that could be a choking hazard for a younger child

Caring for toys

- Check toys regularly and always throw away any broken ones.
- Don't mix old and new batteries. Change them all at the same time, otherwise the strong batteries will make the weak ones very hot.
- Keep toys in a toy box. Toys can bring about accidents or injuries if left on the floor.

Babies and toddlers

- Remove ribbons from a baby's soft toys.
- Check that the eyes, noses, ears, or bells on soft toys and dolls are well secured.
- Attach cot toys with a very short string and remove them as soon as your baby can sit up.
- Remove activity centres or bulky toys from a cot as soon as your child can stand because they provide a foothold for climbing out of the cot.
- Don't let babies chew on furry toys: the fur is a choking hazard.
- Never let a young child play with a toy that is not recommended for his age-group: it may contain small pieces on which he could choke.
- Don't leave baby or toddler to play in a room on his own.
- Do not use baby walkers.

Make sure that toys that increase mobility are stable

Garden

Your garden can be a safe and interesting place for your children to play. Children will find their own corners to play in but you must clear away rubbish and remove obvious hazards:

- Lock gates that lead out of the garden and make sure fences are secure.
- Check garden furniture or play equipment regularly to make sure that it is stable and safe. Site it over grass not paving stones.
- Keep pets off areas where children play.
- Make sure paving is even and remove moss: children may easily trip or slip.

Plants

Many plants are poisonous if eaten and digested in large quantities. Small pieces, or one or two berries, are not fatal but may cause some discomfort and stomach upset.

- Tell your child about the dangers of eating berries, and keep babies and toddlers away from them.
- Remove plants that you know to be poisonous, such as deadly nightshade, laburnum, and toadstools.
- Cut back any prickly plants, such as roses, brambles, and holly. They can give nasty scratches, especially to your or your child's eyes.

Warn your child not to eat berries or leaves

Sheds

These can be exciting dens for children.

- If your shed is full of gardening equipment or tools, tell your child that it is out of bounds, keep it locked at all times, and hide the key.
- Put any chemicals, such as weedkiller or slug pellets, out of reach in containers with safety catches.

Water in the garden

Babies and toddlers are especially at risk if they slip and fall, even in shallow water.

- Never leave children unattended when they are playing in, or near, water.
- Keep ponds covered and fenced off, and cover water butts and empty dustbins that collect rainwater.
- Always empty out a paddling pool when your children have finished playing in it and turn it upside-down in case it rains.

Gardening

- Don't put down chemicals when children will be playing in the garden.
- Don't mow the lawn while children are close by because stone chips may become dislodged and fly up into their eyes.
- Put away all garden tools when you have finished using them.

Check that he is playing in a clean, safe area with safe toys

Garage and car safety

Always leave your garage locked; likewise keep the car locked, even if it is on a driveway off the road or in a garage. Keep the car keys where the children cannot reach them. Don't give the keys to your baby to play with as they are not clean and he could drop them.

Garages

- Keep the garage locked and discourage your child from going in there.
- Keep equipment, chemicals, or tools out of your child's reach and locked away if possible.
- Make sure you know where your child is when you are driving into, or out of, the garage.
- If you keep a deep freeze in the garage, it should be locked at all times.

Cars

- Never leave a young child unattended in a car, even if you can see the car.
- Never let a child sit in the front seat of the car if there is an airbag.
- Don't let your child play with the car windows, whether manual or electric. Windows can trap a child's head or fingers.
- Remove the cigarette lighter from the car altogether.
- Watch out for your child's fingers when you shut the car doors.
- Use child locks on rear doors until your child is at least six years old.
- Teach your child to get out of the car on the pavement side.
- If your child is helping you wash or tidy the car, always make sure you have removed the car keys from the ignition first.

Car seats

Always put your child into a special safety seat when you strap him into the car. Do not buy a second-hand car seat because some car seats are reconditioned after a crash and will not be safe. Choose the correct seat for the weight and development of your child:

Check the seat fixing and baby's straps are securely fastened

- Babies up to 13kg (29lb) – about 12–15 months – should travel in a rear-facing car seat. The baby is harnessed into the seat and the seat is held in place by the car seat belts. The safest place for your baby to travel is on the rear seat of your car. Make sure you do not place your baby in a rear-facing car seat on the front passenger seat if there is an airbag fitted because the impact of an airbag inflating could cause serious injury.
- Never hold a baby on your lap or inside your own seatbelt: he would be thrown out of the car or crushed by your body weight in a crash.
- Older babies and toddlers, up to 18kg (40lb), need a car seat in the back of the car. Some seats have an integral harness for the child, which fits over his shoulders, across his hips, and between his legs. The seats are held in place by the adult seat belt, or straps that you fix into the car. Other types of seat use the adult belt to restrain both the child and the seat. Some new cars have special ISO-fix seat fixings for child car seats.
- Primary school children should travel in a booster seat. Without it, adult seat belts are neither comfortable nor safe: the shoulder part cuts across the child's neck, and the lap strap lies across his stomach, which could cause internal injury in a crash. A booster seat raises a young child so that the shoulder part lies across his upper chest and the lap strap lies across his hips. A lap strap on its own is not sufficient as it does not restrain the child's upper body.

Out and about

After the home, most childhood accidents occur in the street. Teach your child the rules of the road from an early age, reminding him to stay alert for traffic and to cross in a safe place. It takes a long time for children to develop a true road sense.

What a child understands

- Three-year-olds can learn that the pavement is safe and the road is dangerous.
- Five-year-olds can learn how to cross the road, but they are still not able to put this knowledge into practice on their own.
- Eight-year-olds can cross quiet streets on their own, but they are not yet able to judge the speed and distance of traffic.
- Twelve-year-olds can judge the speed of an oncoming car, but are still easily distracted by friends.

Street and road safety

Whenever you are out with your child, show him how to be aware of his own safety.

- When out shopping or walking near a road, use reins or a wrist strap for a toddler, to stop him running off without you.
- Encourage a young child to hold your hand when you are near the road or waiting to cross a road.

Insist that he always wears a protective helmet

Maintain the bike in good working order

Learning how to cross the road

Teach your child the rules of the road:

- Find a safe place to cross, then stop.
- Stand on the pavement, near the kerb.
- Look all around for traffic, and listen.
- If traffic is coming, let it pass.
- When there is no traffic near, walk straight across the road.
- Look and listen for traffic while you cross.

- Teach your child by example and always find a safe place to cross a road. This may be a zebra crossing, a pelican crossing with lights, an underpass, or a footbridge. If there is no designated crossing point, aim for a large gap between parked cars, where you and your child can see a long way in both directions.
- At a zebra crossing teach your child to stop and wait until all the traffic has stopped and to stop at the island halfway across, if there is one.
- When using a pelican crossing at traffic lights, encourage your child to press the button and always wait until the traffic has stopped before crossing.

Bikes

- Children under 10 years old should not cycle on roads in traffic without an adult and all children should have cycle training before going on the road.
- Make sure your child can be seen when he's riding his bike – with bright fluorescent colours by day and reflectors on his clothes and bike by night. He should wear an approved helmet to protect his head.

Where to play

What may seem common sense to you is not obvious to children.

- Show your child where it is safe to play – the playground, or local recreation ground, for example – and supervise him if necessary.
- Teach your child the dangers of playing in open areas, such as roads, building sites, and quarries.
- Tell your child not to play in the street, or on a pavement near the kerb – even if your street is quiet.
- Tell him that he must never chase a ball, a pet, or another child into the road.

Prams and buggies

- Never push a pram or buggy out into the traffic to see if the road is clear to cross. Pull the buggy to one side and check whether the road is safe. Remember that a child's buggy sticks out in front of you by at least 1m (3ft).
- When you park a pram or buggy, put on the brakes and point it away from traffic.
- Never tie your dog to the pram.
- Never leave a baby unattended.

Harness your baby into his buggy

In the playground

All playgrounds should comply with safety standards; report any faulty equipment to your local authority.

- The play area must be safely fenced off and away from roads.
- There should be a soft, even surface, such as bark chippings or rubber tiles, around equipment.
- Slides should be no higher than 2.4m (8ft) and preferably constructed on an earth mound to break any falls.
- Roundabouts should be low, with a smooth surface, designed so that young children can't get their feet stuck underneath.
- Climbing frames should be no higher than 2.4m (8ft), completely stable, and built over sand or a very soft surface to break falls.
- Swings for young children must have safety guards.
- There should be a clearly defined play area for toddlers and young children, set away from the more boisterous activities of older children.
- There should be someone to contact if any of the equipment is faulty.
- Dogs must not be allowed inside playgrounds.

Check that swings are set apart from main play equipment

> **❗ IMPORTANT**
>
> - Remind your child of the dangers of talking to strangers. Have a code word that a friend can use if colllecting your child. Tell your child not to go with anybody unless they use the code.

Travelling with babies and children

Away from your home all the same rules of safety apply. However, you should be aware that the place you are staying in would not necessarily have been planned with young children in mind.

- If there is a swimming pool, never leave your child unattended in or near the water and, if there is a fence around it, keep the gate shut.
- Take baby milk and/or food with you as your child may not like what is available locally.

Travelling abroad

- Make sure your child's immunisations are up to date. Some countries recommend additional vaccination, or anti-malaria medication; ask when booking a trip.
- Don't forget to take the necessary paperwork; babies and children need their own passports for most countries. It is a good idea to keep a photocopy of each passport (yours as well) in a separate bag.
- If you are hiring a car, always ask for child safety seats, or take your child's car seat with you.
- Make sure hire cars are fitted with sufficient safety belts and check that they are in good condition (not frayed) and working properly.
- Take insect repellent suitable for babies and young children, as they are particularly susceptible to insect bites. Apply the repellant in the early evening and again at bedtime when the insects are most active.
- Wash vegetables, salads, and fruit in cooled, boiled water or bottled water if there is any doubt about the local water.
- Boil water used to make up baby foods or milk.

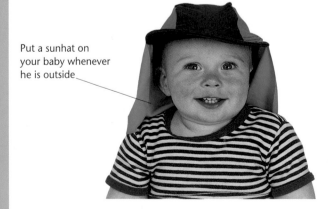

Put a sunhat on your baby whenever he is outside

Air travel

- If booking tickets for children under the age of two, ask for seats where you can use a child safety seat or a sky cot.
- Give your baby a breastfeed, bottlefeed, or a dummy to suck as the plane ascends and descends because the change in pressure can cause earache in babies and children. Give an older child a sweet to suck, but make sure he does not choke on it.
- Take any food or milk that a baby needs on the journey. Airlines don't generally carry baby food, though they can often heat food or milk for you.
- Give your baby or child plenty to drink during the flight, to prevent dehydration.

Sun protection

- Use sun block that protects your child from ultra violet A rays (UVA) and ultra violet B rays (UVB). The sun protector factor (SPF) numbers relate to UVA – chose SPF 30 – and a star-rating system indicates UVB protection. Re-apply regularly, especially after he has been in water. Use a cream that you know your child is not allergic to.
- Keep your baby or child's arms and legs covered as much as possible. Dress him in clothes made of closely woven fabric made of natural fibres.
- Make sure your child is protected by the shade in the middle of the day (about 10am until 4pm).
- Put a wide-brimmed hat on your child's head that covers his neck and face and use a parasol on a buggy.
- Give your child plenty to drink to prevent dehydration. If you are breastfeeding offer your baby more feeds; give a bottlefed baby plain water.

Index

A

B

C

Acknowledgments

Dorling Kindersley would like to thank:
Joe Mulligan, Head of First Aid Services, the British Red Cross, for his help with the photography; Cardiac Science Corporation for the loan of the paediatric defibrillator; the Child Accident Prevention Trust (www.capt.org.uk) for reviewing *Child Safety*; Constance Novis for proofreading; Hilary Bird for the index; the following for modelling:
Children Aleena Awan, Navaz Awan, Max Buckingham, Madeline Cameron, Alfie Clarke, Amy Davies, Thomas Davies, James Dow, Kyla Edwards, Austin Enil, Lia Foa, Maya Foa, Jessica Forge, Kashi Gorton, Emily Gorton, Thomas Greene, Alexander Harrison, Rupert Harrison, Ben Harrison, Jessica Harris-Voss, Hannah Headam, Jake Hutton, Rosemary Kaloki, Winnie Kaloki, Ella Kaye, Maddy Kaye, Jade Lamb, Emily Leney, Crispin Lord, Daniel Lord, Harriet Lord, Ailsa McCaughrean, Fiona Maine, Tom Maine, Kincaid Malik-White, Maija Marsh, Oliver Metcalf, Eloise Morgan, Tom Razazan, Jimmy Razazan, Georgia Ritter, Rebecca Sharples, Ben Sharples, Thomas Sharples, Ben Walker, Robyn Walker, Amy Beth Walton Evans, Hanna Warren-Green, Simon Weekes, Joseph Weir, Lily Ziegler.
Adults Shaila Awan, Claire le Bas, Joanna Benwell, Angela Cameron, Georgina Davies, Marion Davies, Sophie Dow, Tina Edwards, Rachel Fitchett, Emma Foa, Emma Forge, Caroline Greene, Susan Harrison, Victoria Harrison, Julia Harris-Voss, Roy Headam, Emma Hutton, Helga Lien Evans, Sylvie Jordan, Jane Kaloki, David Kaye, Louise Kaye, Philip Lord, Geraldine McCaughrean, Diana Maine, Brian Marsh, Jonathan Metcalf, Francoise Morgan, Juliette Norsworthy, Anna Pizzi, Hossein Razazan, Angela Sharples, John Sharples, Miranda Tunbridge, Vanessa Walker, Catherine Warren-Green, Toni Weekes, Robert Ziegler.

Make-up: Wendy Holmes, Pebbles, Geoff Portas

Additional photographs Andy Crawford, Steve Gorton, Ray Mollers, Suzannah Price, Dave Rudkin, Steve Shott

Emergency contact details

IN AN EMERGENCY GO TO THE NEAREST TELEPHONE
AND DIAL 999. ASK FOR THE POLICE, AMBULANCE
OR FIRE BRIGADE

FOR EMERGENCY MEDICAL ADVICE CALL NHS
DIRECT TELEPHONE 0845 4647

Doctor
Name: _____
Address: _____
_____
Telephone: _____
Surgery Hours: _____

Health Visitor
Name: _____
Clinic Address: _____
_____
Telephone: _____
Clinic Hours: _____

Dentist
Name: _____
Address: _____
_____
Telephone: _____
Surgery Hours: _____

Hospital Accident & Emergency
Address: _____
_____
Telephone: _____

Late Night Chemist
Address: _____
_____

Local Police Station
Telephone: _____

Gas Emergency Service
Telephone: _____

Electricity Emergency Service
Telephone: _____

Water Emergency Service
Telephone: _____

British Red Cross

The British Red Cross runs first aid courses for all ages. For further
information, get in touch with your local British Red Cross office; you will
find the number in the telephone directory or in the Yellow Pages.
Alternatively, visit www.redcross.org.uk.

British Red Cross, UK Office
44 Moorfields, London, EC2Y 9AL
Telephone: 0870 170 7000

The Red Cross emblem is a symbol of protection during armed conflicts,
and its use is restricted by law.

Details of the royalties
payable to the British Red
Cross can be obtained by
writing to the publisher
Dorling Kindersley at the
following address:
80 Strand
London
WC2R 0RL